HIGHLIGHTS ON HEMODYNAMICS

Edited by **Theodoros Aslanidis**

Highlights on Hemodynamics
http://dx.doi.org/10.5772/intechopen.73803
Edited by Theodoros Aslanidis

Contributors

Olena Ivanivna Lutsenko, Branislav Kolarovszki, Yoko Kato, Gaiping Zhao, Theodoros Aslanidis

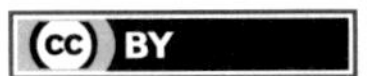

Notice

Statements and opinions expressed in the chapters are these of the individual contributors and not necessarily those of the editors or publisher. No responsibility is accepted for the accuracy of information contained in the published chapters. The publisher assumes no responsibility for any damage or injury to persons or property arising out of the use of any materials, instructions, methods or ideas contained in the book.

First published in London, United Kingdom, 2018 by IntechOpen
IntechOpen is the global imprint of INTECHOPEN LIMITED, registered in England and Wales, registration number: 11086078, The Shard, 25th floor, 32 London Bridge Street
London, SE19SG – United Kingdom
Printed in Croatia

British Library Cataloguing-in-Publication Data
A catalogue record for this book is available from the British Library

Additional hard copies can be obtained from orders@intechopen.com

Highlights on Hemodynamics, Edited by Theodoros Aslanidis
p. cm.
Print ISBN 978-1-78923-793-1
Online ISBN 978-1-78923-794-8

For EU product safety concerns:
IN TECH d.o.o., Prolaz Marije Krucifikse Kozulić 3, 51000 Rijeka, Croatia, info@intechopen.com or visit our website at intechopen.com.

Meet the editor

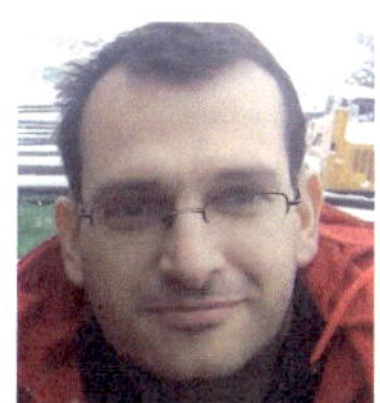

Dr. Theodoros K. Aslanidis received his Doctor of Medicine degree from the Plovdiv Medical University, Bulgaria, and his PhD degree from the Aristotle University of Thessaloniki, Greece. After serving in the Hellenic Army Force as a medical doctor, he worked as a rural physician at the Outhealth Centre, Iraklia and Serres' General Hospital, Greece. He completed his residency in Anaesthesiology at "Hippokratio" General Hospital of Thessaloniki, followed by fellowship training in Critical Care at AHEPA University Hospital and a postgraduate program in Prehospital Emergency Medicine. He served as an EMS Physician and Emergency Communication Centre Medic at the Hellenic National Centre for Emergency Care before moving to his current post as consultant-researcher at the Intensive Care Unit of St. Paul General Hospital of Thessaloniki, Greece. His research interests are medical writing, data analysis, critical emergency medicine, neurosonology and electrodermal activity.

Contents

Preface

Hemodynamics is an essential link between cardiovascular anatomy and cardiovascular physiology. Clear understanding of the physical factors that govern blood movement in the cardiovascular system is a necessary prerequisite for clinical medicine. Yet, the complexity and the unique character of the human body and the changes that occur during various pathological states make this task extremely difficult.

Thus, it is not a surprise that almost six centuries after Leonardo da Vinci's first hemodynamic observations, the interest and research about hemodynamics are continuing to grow.

We have moved from simple macroscopic observations to computational modeling, functional hemodynamic monitoring and the relation of hemodynamics and hemorheology. Current research of pathophysiological changes at both the microscopic and macroscopic levels "unlocks" new knowledge every day.

Within this frame, the current book published by InTechOpen® focuses on hemodynamic issues of special interest. The authors offer the readers not only a "vigorous" review of the current literature but also a research direction full of promises for further advancement.

Dr. Theodoros Aslanidis
Intensive Care Unit
St. Paul General Hospital of Thessaloniki
Greece

Section 1

Introduction

Chapter 1

Introductory Chapter: Hemodynamic Management. The Problem of Monitoring Choice

Theodoros Aslanidis

Additional information is available at the end of the chapter

http://dx.doi.org/10.5772/intechopen.79931

1. Introduction

Technology progress has given us the opportunity to monitor almost every aspect of the cardiovascular system down to the level of tissue microcirculation. However, the choice of the right tool is often a challenge, depending both on institutional capabilities (availability of the device) and on operator training. The present chapter consists a short literature review about the subject.

It is more than three centuries that Reverend Stephen Hales have made the first invasive measurement of blood pressure and cardiac output [1]. During that time, there has been a tremendous progress both in hemodynamics physiology and pathophysiology understanding and in modes of cardiovascular monitoring. Today, it is considered basic and essential knowledge for every physician. The paradox: the more we know about cardiovascular circulation, the more we understand our ignorance. The present chapter focuses on some of the problems encountered during hemodynamic monitoring.

2. Describing the challenges

Current technology provides us with a vast range of tools for hemodynamic evaluation. Yet, whether it uses an invasive technique or not, performs one or more calculations provides with discrete or continuous data, seem to have minor importance. As any tool, we need to know its limitations and choose carefully. Vincent et al. [2] attempted to suggest the key principles of hemodynamic monitoring. The most important of them:

1. No hemodynamic monitoring technique can improve outcome by itself.
2. Monitoring requirements may very over time. Moreover, the highly depend on the availability of the devices and the training of the operators.

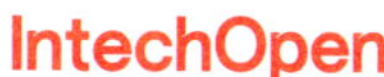

3. There are no optimal hemodynamic parameters for every patient.
4. We need to combine and integrate variables.
5. Continuous measurements are preferable.
6. Non-invasiveness is not the only issue.
7. Cardiac output is estimated not measured.

Chan and Khan [3] reviewed the problem from a more physiological point of view. They claimed that since there is no hemodynamic monitoring that can provide us data for the "whole" cardiovascular system and that the main role of the latter is oxygen delivery, we need to choose our monitoring according to the target part of the cardiovascular system and to aim at correlation of the data with oxygen delivery. Thus, we might have a better connection between monitoring and outcome.

Another issue brought up by Peter et al. [4, 5], is calibration. There are calibrated and non-calibrated techniques for hemodynamic monitoring. Though calibrated (invasive in the majority of them) methods seem to work better in unstable patients, careful interpretation of the provided data is needed. On the other hand, as new technology is integrated in medical devices, the future seems to belong to non-invasive techniques.

And what about continuity of data and of care? For example, pulmonary artery catheter (PAC), which triggered a boom in hemodynamic monitoring, provides only static variables. A snapshot of patient's status, often not enough to determine the right therapeutic strategy. Along with that if the same patient is admitted to Emergency Department with an A hemodynamic profile derived from arterial pressure wave, transported to ward where he had a B profile measured via suprasternal Doppler and ended in ICU where PAC and bio-impedance measurements are available, do we take in mind the previous profiles (A and B) or not? One option is to reject previous measurements, thus risking loosing valuable data. Another option is to just average measurements. However, plans based on average assumptions, are on average wrong.

The latter is even more valid for the therapeutic strategy that we may choose. If a drug causes on average an increase in cardiac output (CO), how do we know that our patient lies within this average?

The previous problem is perplexed by the fact that different modes of monitoring may provide us with different variables. CO may be a common parameter for various devices, yet extra lung water index, oxygen extraction ration, wedge pulmonary pressure, peak velocity and Doppler driven dp/dt may be harder to combine.

3. Solution

The aforementioned create a puzzle to solve each time a physician decides that hemodynamic monitoring is needed.

Monitoring that combines conditions and advantages of each monitoring technique could be a solution to the problem. Thus, for example CO based on partial CO_2 rebreathing is considered less reliable in cases of respiratory failure [2, 6], right ventricular failure or tricuspid regurgitation may compromise PAC derived measurement of CO [7], Doppler flow studies focusing on the descending thoracic aorta may not provide a reliable measurement of the total cardiac output (for example, with epidural use), and are invalid in the presence of intra-aortic balloon pumping [6]. CO measurements derived from peripheral arterial pressure waveform have shown luck of accuracy in patients with intracerebral hemorrhage [8], functional hemodynamic parameters like pulse pressure variation or stroke volume variation need regular sinus rhythm, etc.

As a consequence, several reports tried to suggest guidelines for hemodynamic monitoring in specific conditions, like for example, circulatory shock [9], sepsis [10], or patients under thoracic anesthesia [11].

Personalized hemodynamic monitoring concept emerges as the best available option. This is a very difficult task in most cases, as it assumes the existence of a dynamic close loop system with constantly new hemodynamic targets – adjusted to specific patient within a given clinical and time frame [12, 13].

Yet, even though we cannot form an individualized guideline, ongoing research, both clinical, experimental (including computational modeling of cardiovascular system and simulation of different pathological conditions) will help us create and clarify the exact theoretic concept which will direct the management. Along with that, formation of clear institutional policy about both the availability and the training of the personnel of each healthcare facility are needed, in order to standardize and regulate the use of certain medical devices over others (within the institution).

Conflict of interests

The author has no conflict of interest.

Author details

Theodoros Aslanidis

Address all correspondence to: thaslan@hotmail.com

Intensive Care Unit, St. Paul General Hospital of Thessaloniki, Greece

References

[1] Nossaman BD, Scruggs BA, Nossaman VE, Murthy SN, Kadowitz PJ. History of right heart catheterization: 100 years of experimentation and methodology development. Cardiology in Review. 2010;**18**(2):94-101. DOI: 10.1097/CRD.0b013e3181ceff67

[2] Vincent JL, Rhodes A, Perel A, Martin GS, Della Rocca G, Vallet B, Pinsky MR, Hofer CK, Teboul JL, de Boode WP, Scolletta S, Vieillard-Baron A, De Backer D, Walley KR, Maggiorini M, Singer M. Update on hemodynamic monitoring—A consensus of 16. Critical Care. 2011;**15**(4):229. DOI: 10.1186/cc10291

[3] Chan YK, Khan ZH. Hemodynamic monitoring—A physiological appraisal. Acta Anaesthesiologica Taiwanica. 2011;**49**(4):154-158. DOI: 10.1016/j.aat.2011.11.002

[4] Peeters Y, Bernards J, Mekeirele M, Hoffmann B, De Raes M, Malbrain ML. Hemodynamic monitoring: To calibrate or not to calibrate? Part 1–Calibrated techniques. Anaesthesiology Intensive Therapy. 2015;**47**(5):487-500. DOI: 10.5603/AIT.a2015.0073

[5] Bernards J, Mekeirele M, Hoffmann B, Peeters Y, De Raes M, Malbrain ML. Hemodynamic monitoring: To calibrate or not to calibrate? Part 2–Non-calibrated techniques. Anaesthesiology Intensive Therapy. 2015;**47**(5):501-516. DOI: 10.5603/AIT.a2015.0076

[6] Ramsingh D, Alexander B, Cannesson M. Clinical review: Does it matter which hemodynamic monitoring system is used? Critical Care. 2013;**17**(2):208. DOI: 10.1186/cc11814

[7] Ho KM. Pitfalls of hemodynamic monitoring in postoperative and critical setting. Anaesthesia and Intensive Care. 2016;**44**(1):14-19

[8] Junttila EK, Koskenkari JK, Ohtonen PP, Ala-Kokko TI. Uncalibrated arterial pressure waveform analysis for cardiac output monitoring is biased by low peripheral resistance in patients with intracranial haemorrhage. British Journal of Anaesthesia. 2011;**107**:581-586. DOI: 10.1093/bja/aer170

[9] Cecconi M, De Backer D, Antonelli M, Beale R, Bakker J, Hofer C, Jaeschke R, Mebazaa A, Pinsky MR, Teboul JL, Vincent JL, Rhodes A. Consensus on circulatory shock and hemodynamic monitoring. Task force of the European Society of intensive care medicine. Intensive Care Medicine. 2014;**40**(12):1795-1815. DOI: 10.1007/s00134-014-3525-z

[10] Cecconi M, Arulkumaran N, Kilic J, Ebm C, Rhodes A. Update on hemodynamic monitoring and management in septic patients. Minerva Anestesiologica. 2014;**80**(6):701-711

[11] Hofer CK, Rex S, Ganter MT. Update on minimally invasive hemodynamic monitoring in thoracic anesthesia. Current Opinion in Anaesthesiology. 2014;**27**(1):28-35. DOI: 10.1097/ACO.0000000000000034

[12] Su LX, Liu DW. Personalized hemodynamic therapy concept for shock resuscitation. Chinese Medical Journal. 2018;**131**:1240-1243. DOI: 10.4103/0366-6999.231511

[13] Saugel B, Vincent JL, Wagner JY. Personalized hemodynamic management. Current Opinion in Critical Care. 2017;**23**:334-341. DOI: 10.1097/MCC.0000000000000422

Section 2

Special topics

Chapter 2

Functioning of the Cardiovascular System of Women in Different Phases of the Ovarian-Menstrual Cycle

Olena Lutsenko

Additional information is available at the end of the chapter

http://dx.doi.org/10.5772/intechopen.79633

Abstract

Seventy seven women with 17–19 years of age examined central hemodynamics and its wave structure at rest, with orthopedic and psychoemotional load in different phases of the ovarian cycle (OC). It was established that in the luteal phase of the OC in the lying position, the blood pressure was higher than in other phases. In orthoprost in the luteal phase, in comparison with other phases, the growth of cardiac rhythm wave strength in the range of 0.04–0.15 Hz is observed, their concentration and connection with oscillations of the shock volume of blood, and the leveling of differences in blood pressure levels. The involvement of spontaneous baro-reflex sensitivity of the studied states and reactions is discussed.

Keywords: central hemodynamics, variability of the cardiac rhythm, women, ovarian-menstrual cycle

1. Introduction

The basis of modern human physiology is the systematic approach, the synthesis of the theory of functional systems and the theory of adaptation, which allows us to obtain meaningful information about the functional state of the organism during ontogenesis and use the obtained data for practical actions [1–3].

Heart rate variability (HRV) is a fundamental physiological property of the human body, which reflects the state of regulatory mechanisms of homeostasis, in particular, the tone of the autonomic nervous system [4]. Therefore, the study of HRV has become important for qualitative diagnosis, prediction, and prevention of various diseases [5, 6].

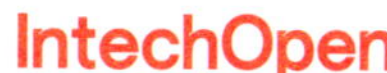

At the beginning of the twenty-first century, the attention of researchers is drawn to the study of the variability of the duration of the interval R-R [7–10], blood pressure [11–13], shock volume [14], respiratory arrhythmia [15–17], and the relationship of wave changes in various hemodynamic parameters. This is due to the wide introduction of information technology to the theory and practice of medicine and physiology, high diagnostic value of parameters of regulatory rhythms of hemodynamics.

Of all the physiological systems of humans, the most important and little studied is reproductive [18–22]. In particular, insufficient research on the chronostructure of physiological systems in women suggests that the productivity and stability of body systems, in addition to the annual seasonal changes in various physiological functions and the seasonal exacerbation of some diseases, significantly affect the ovarian-menstrual cycle [23, 24].

An analysis of the above-mentioned developments of scientists and practitioners shows that the preservation and strengthening of health significantly depends on the further study of adaptive reactions of the female body, taking into account the ovarian-menstrual cycle, the individual annual, and the seasonal period of physiological functions.

On the adaptive trophic role of the sympathetic department of the VNS, including the reproduction, one of the first pointed academician Orbeli [15]. However, to date, the question of the state of the autonomic nervous system, including the activity of the cardiac rhythm, in women during the menstrual cycle is inadequate. A series of review papers [25–27] provides data on age and gender changes in some HRV indicators. However, these data relate, preferably, to short (2–5 min.) Records of R-R intervals are performed on contingents of persons with different pathologies [28–30]. At the same time, the characteristics of the wave structure of the vibrations of hemodynamic indices in healthy women in different physiological conditions and loads in the process of ontogenesis are insufficiently analyzed.

It should be emphasized the existence of certain contradictions in the results of various studies of the variability of the cardiac rhythm in women in different phases of the ovarian-menstrual cycle and the treatment of their mechanisms.

There remains an inadequate study of the problem associated with the influence of the ovarian-menstrual cycle on the indicators of central hemodynamics and cardiac rhythm variability under different physiological conditions. In particular, studies of changes in the oscillations of the shock volume of blood, spontaneous baro-reflex sensitivity in women under different stresses.

In Ketel et al. conducted in randomized tubes for 149 men and 137 middle-aged women, revealed that HRV levels were inversely related to age and heart rate in both sexes. The level of LF in men is significantly higher than in women and is negatively related to the level of triglycerides, insulin. The power of the R-R interval for women is higher than that of men.

The widespread introduction of the ECG holter monitoring method into clinical practice allowed the evaluation of HRV in the course of the day and at certain intervals, and also used this method for studying the state of autonomic regulation of the heart rate. Extreme values of total spectrum power and power in the very low and low frequency range under holter monitoring of women in comparison with men were also recorded in Fluckiger et al. [31].

In this case, the power in the ranges of low and high frequencies was negatively correlated with age. The total power of the spectrum was relatively reduced between 20–29 years and 60–69 years by 30%.

The same gender and age characteristics of the wave structure of the heart rate were also confirmed in measurements of 302 men and 312 women conducted by Bai et al., for 653 persons performed by Aubert et al. [7], and on 276 persons conducted by Barrett et al. The gender differences in HRV are measured at the sixth decade of the human life cycle. Changes in the cardiac rhythm and its spectral components during orthopedic trial at this age did not have sexual differences.

There are significant differences in the reactivity of fluctuations in the interval of R-R and the peripheral pressure of men and women on physical, mental, and cold loads. So in the research of Peshakova [32] shows that women under these conditions have a greater centralization of the mechanisms of regulation of the cardiovascular system, and for men, an increase in the activity of the sympathetic link of the autonomic nervous system.

Many researchers [33–36] point out that cardiovascular analysis is more appropriate to detect minor fluctuations of the VNS activity during the menstrual cycle than the use of traditional indicators such as heart rate and arterial pressure. However, the results of studies of changes in the heart rate in different phases of the menstrual cycle are still controversial. It should be noted that significant changes in HRV in women of reproductive age, both at rest and during psychoemotional stresses, may be due to the phase of the ovarian cycle [37–42]. SDNN in young women was the highest during the follicular phase of the menstrual cycle [43]. According to Koening and co-authors [44], in women during the luteal phase compared with the follicular showed an increase in the activity of the sympathetic department of the autonomic autonomy of the autonomy according to the HRV indices. However, a group of researchers, Grossman et al. [45], insists on the absence of differences in the parameters of the wave structure of blood pressure and heart rate when performing orthopedic and stimulating carotid sinus in women in different phases of the ovarian cycle.

Japanese scientists [43] demonstrate a significant increase in sympathetic and decreased parasympathetic activity in the lutein phase compared to follicular, as evidenced by an increase in the values of LF/HF and LF, as well as a decrease in HF in the luteal phase. The facts of the increase in the level of LF/HF in the early and middle luteal phase are given in Holzen et al. [46], with the late luteal phase showing a tendency to decrease the level of LF/HF. At the same time, some researchers, Princi et al. [47] and Sato et al. [39] refute this assumption, indicating that there is no significant change.

Although some researchers point to an increase in the level of HF in the follicular phase compared with the luteal and menstrual phase, measurements were made only one [48–50] or twice a week [51] during the cycle. Since hormonal and physiological changes during the menstrual cycle are complex and complex, they can not be characterized by two measurements, which indicate the need for long-term research.

In studies [52], in 10 completely healthy women, it was found that spontaneous baroreflectory sensitivity increases during the luteal phase compared to the follicular phase. It was stated that there were certain differences in the logRSA fluctuations during the menstrual cycle, which were related to the average NSC indexes.

According to Weisman, there are significant changes in both the wave structure of the cardiac rhythm and its reactivity to the burden on women in the first 20 weeks of pregnancy. So, normally in this period, the power of OT components increases, often the synchronization of respiratory and baroreflector waves is observed. In pathological development of pregnancy, there is an inversion of such regulatory relations.

The variability of the cardiac rhythm during the physiological course of pregnancy is reduced, which indicates an increase in the activity of the sympathetic department of the autonomic nervous system [21, 53]. In women with gestosis, HRV is more pronounced. Revealed by scientists, the facts of changes in HRV with other hypertensive states in pregnant women, as well as in normal and complicated childbirth are few and controversial. The emphasis is placed on the prospect of further study of sympathetic activity in relation to changes in HRV in pregnant and childbearing, as well as on the need for widespread introduction of cardiointervalography in obstetrics.

The process of reproduction in humans regulates complex neuroendocrine mechanisms, so the normal functioning of the reproductive system is possible only with the integrated control of the nervous and humoral signals. One of the manifestations of complex changes in the body of a woman is the menstrual cycle: cyclic changes in the hypothalamus, pituitary gland, and ovaries; cyclic changes in the target organs (uterus, fallopian tubes, vagina, and mammary glands); cyclic changes in the endocrine, nervous, and other systems of the organism. The most pronounced changes occur in the ovaries (ripening of the follicles, ovulation, and development of the yellow body) and the uterus (desquamation of the endometrium is actually menstruation, regeneration and proliferation of the functional layer, secretory changes in it, and again desquamation). Due to these changes, the reproductive function of the woman is carried out: ovulation, fertilization, implantation, and development of the embryo in the uterus. If implantation does not occur, pregnancy does not occur, and the functional layer of the endometrium is exfoliated, from the genital tract, there is a spotting (menstruation). The appearance of menstrual discharge indicates the completion of cyclical changes in the body and the absence of pregnancy. The main symptom of normal functioning of the reproductive system of a woman is a normal menstrual cycle. This biorhythm is genetically determined in a healthy woman, and it is stable throughout the generative age according to its parameters.

2. Methods

Seventy seven women aged 18–19 were tested under the conditioned close to the state of basal metabolism in the prone position, at tilt test, and during the test of psychic-emotional stress (Makarenko) [54]. As a mental load, we used a 10-minute test to determine the performance of the brain in the feedback mode by the method of prof. M.V. Makarenko using the Diagnostic-1 system. Each woman was tested three times: in follicular phase (I), ovulation (II), and luteal phase (III) of ovarian-menstrual cycle. Cycle phases were determined according to anamnesis, taking basal body temperature, and using a set of inkjet ovulation tests "Solo" (IND Diagnostic, Inc., Canada).

The main method for determining the phases of the CMC was the collection of anamnesis. Using the test-microscope "Arbor" in the studied group of students examined the presence of ovulation by the nature of the crystallization of saliva. The method is based on the fact that during ovulation, when the concentration of estrogen in the blood of a woman becomes maximal, in saliva, the concentration of salts increases, which is manifested in the maximum crystallization of saliva. Thus, a graphic image on a glass under a microscope was called a "leaf of ferns" (**Figure 1**).

Confirmation of reliability of phase change of the cycle (selectively) was carried out by means of ultrasound diagnostics, the apparatus, HDI 1500, as well as the set of jet tests SoloTM (company "Pharmaco", the registration certificate of the Ministry of Health of Ukraine NO 1856/2003 of 16.05.2008, the international certificate of quality ISO 9001/ISO 13485, and Manufacturer of IND Canada) to determine the ovulation.

The confirmation of the MC phase was also carried out using the technique of basal body temperature measurement Krupko-Bolshova (1986). During the ripening of the egg in the follicular phase of the cycle, against the background of increased estrogen BBT is low (36–37°C), after ovulation, in the lutein phase, begins the temperature increase (37.2–38°C), which is due to the low estrogen levels in the background of increased progesterone in the blood of women.

BBT was measured every morning, at the same time, from 600 to 800 hours (depending on the time of year), not getting out of bed for 5 minutes, mercury thermometer in the rectum at a depth of about 5 cm. Rozultaty entered into the table: date, day of the cycle, BT, and special circumstances.

The difference between the mean values of the second and first phase of the CTD can be 0.5–0.8°C, but it should not be less than 0.4–0.50°C. This is evidence of the normal course of CMC. If during the whole cycle the temperature on the graph is kept, for example, on the same level, or the graph looks like "tyna" (when the low temperature constantly changes high), rather than biphasic, this is due to the fact that ovulation was not (**Figure 2**).

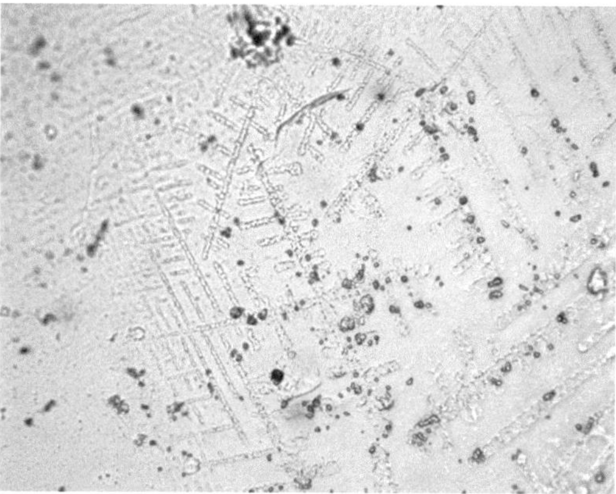

Figure 1. Photo of smear of saliva of student L. (during ovulation).

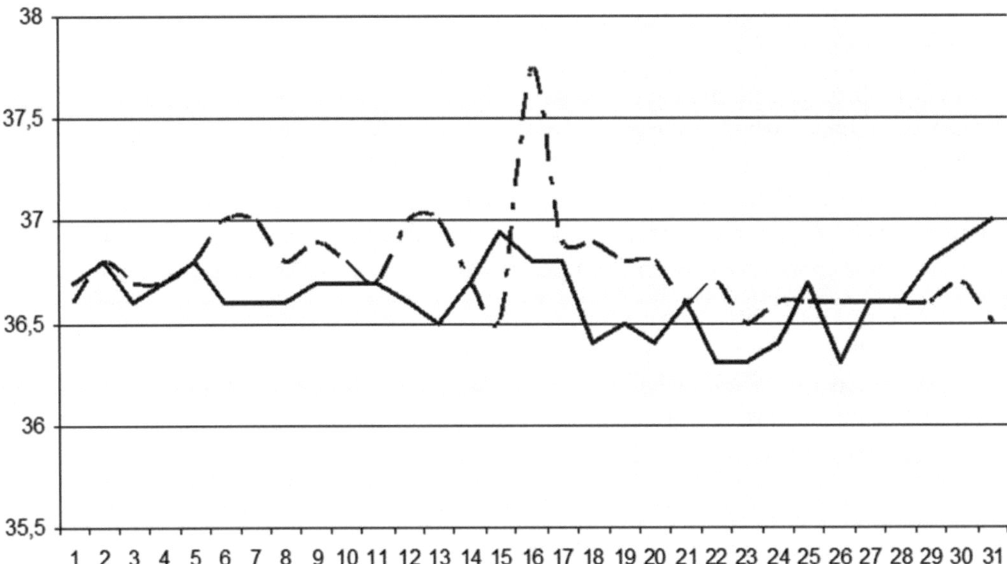

Figure 2. In the middle of the chart changes in basal body temperature in a normal ovarian-menstrual cycle (dashed line) and an anulatory (solid line).

3. Analytical methods

Systolic and diastolic AP (APs and APd, respectively) were measured with Korotkov auscultation method by mercury tonometer ("Riester", Germany). Mean arterial pressure (APm) was calculated with Hickam formula; blood struck volume (BSV) with Kubichek formula [55] by the signals of differentiated impedance rheogram by all the realizations (beat-to-beat) during 5 minutes.

With the help of a rheographer and pneumograph, only cardiointervalograms and pnevmograms were recorded. Cardiointervalograms were recorded using Caspico [56] in MS DOS mode. For this, a cardiac sensor T31 (Polar Electro OU, Finland) was applied to the thoracic cell, which formed 8 ms pulses at the top of the QRS complex. These impulses were telemetrically perceived by the pulse meter A1 and, together with the pnevmogram signal, were transmitted to a 5 kV galvanic switch comparator, which closed the contacts on the LPT port of the computer. The program scanned the device with a frequency of 1000 times per second. The power of R-R and BSV oscillations spectrum was calculated in standard frequency ranges of very low frequencies of 0–0.04 Hz (VLF), low frequencies of 0.04–0.15 Hz (LF), high frequencies of 0.15–0.4 Hz (HF), general oscillation power of 0–0.4 Hz (TP), and normalized power in the range of 0.15–0.4 Hz (HFnorm). Besides, spectral and cross-spectral density and the frequency of the highest amplitude oscillation peak of t-R-R and BSV in the LF range were estimated in the prone position at rest for 5 minute records, at tilt test from the 2nd till the 5th minute and in psycho-emotional test from the 3rd till 7th minute [10].

The method of impedance reopeltysmography was used to calculate cardiac output [57], associated with it indicators of relative blood flow to the body of the chest.

Signals of differentiated ECG and rheograms were fixed with the aid of a biopower RA-5-01 (Kyiv Research Institute of Radio-measuring Equipment). The spring electrodes of rheograms were standardized [10]. The frequency of the reagent's probe signal was 70 kHz.

The pnevmogram signal was obtained from a piezoelectric sensor placed directly in front of the subject (nostrils of the nose).

All these signals were "digitized" through an analog-to-digital converter ADC-1280 (Holit Data Systems, Kiev) with a sampling rate of 860 times per second. The digital signals were stored on the hard disk of the computer for further processing. To analyze signals, identify critical points on them, and export them to spreadsheets, Bioscan [10] was used.

4. Statistical methods

Due to the abnormality of the value distribution of oscillation power of haemodynamic indicators, their medians, the limits of 25 and 75 percentile were found; the average values and their errors for AP indicators distributed normally were determined. The reliability of differences between values in different OMC phases was estimated by means of Wilcoxon paired comparison and Student's t-test. The relationship between indicators was calculated by the nonparametric Spearman correlation coefficient.

5. Results

It was established that in the state of rest in women significant differences between the indices of central hemodynamics, which were analyzed depending on the phases of the CMC, were mostly not observed. However, differences were available at the levels of ATs, ATSer, and ZPO. Changes in these indices were observed in the III phase of the OC ($p < 0.05$) in comparison with the I and II phases (**Table 1**), which is consistent with the results of many authors' studies.

With regulated breathing 6 times/min, we observe the natural increase of practically all indicators in the III phase ($p < 0.05$) in comparison with the I and II phases, except for clinical symptoms, heart rate, CI, and R-R.

When moving to a vertical position in all conditions, there is a natural decrease ($p < 0.001$) of t-R-R, SI, SOC, and increase in LPA (**Table 2**).

Reactivity of blood pressure indicators depended on the OC phase. Thus, in the 1st and 2nd phases, there was a probable increase in ATs, ATD, ATSer, and in III, changes were not statistically significant. This led to the fact that the differences in the levels of ATs and ATSer between the phases of the OC are at rest lying leveling, and there were differences for t-RR between III and I and II phases (676 ± 17, 641 ± 16, 634 ± 11 ms, $p < 0.05$, respectively).

Indicator	Phases of the cycle		
	I	II	III
APs, mm Hg. Art.	98.1 3 ± 1.43	99.22 ± 1.54	101.41 ± 1.87*
APd, mm Hg. Art.	64.38 ± 1.14	65.31 ± 1.05	66.88 ± 1.47
APm, mm Hg. Art.	75.63 ± 1.17	76.61 ± 1.02	78.39 ± 1.48*
т-R-R, ms	801 ± 15.6	784 ± 17.3	803 ± 17.9
SOK, ml	54.96 ± 2.12	58.15 ± 2.93	54.50 ± 2.29
CI, ms	3260 ± 106	3109 ± 87	3304 ± 128
ZPO, din* cm^{-1} *p-5	1569 ± 91	1418 ± 72	1638 ± 82#

*–$p < 0.05$ in comparison with indicators in phase I.
#–$p < 0.05$ in between the indices in the 2nd and 3rd phases.

Table 1. Indicators of central hemodynamics are at rest lying in different phases of the biological cycle of women.

Indicator	Phases of the cycle		
	I	II	III
APs, mm Hg. Art.	98.28 ± 1.46	97.81 ± 1.50	99.37 ± 1.82#
APd, mm Hg. Art.	63.59 ± 0.9	63.90 ± 0.86	66.87 ± 1.34#
APm, mm Hg. Art.	75.15 ± 0.9	75.20 ± 0.95	77.70 ± 1.34#
BS	22.75 ± 0.85	22.29 ± 0.85	22.57 ± 0.85
ZPO, din* cm^{-1} *p-5	1558 ± 71	1458 ± 90*	1591 ± 62#
MVB, ml/min	4051 ± 157	4304 ± 202*	4042 ± 149#
Heart rate ubs/min	75.13 ± 1,29	77.42 ± 1,65*	76.33 ± 1.52
CI, ml	2542 ± 99	2699 ± 127*	2533 ± 92
R-R, ms	805 ± 13	785 ± 16*	796 ± 16

*–$p < 0.05$ in comparison with indicators in phase I.
#–$p < 0.05$ in between the indices in the 2nd and 3rd phases.

Table 2. Indicators of central hemodynamics at regulated respiration (6 times/min) in different phases of the biological cycle.

The reactivity of all indicators in regulated breathing significantly changed in the III phase compared with the 1st and 2nd phases. No changes occurred in the significance of ATs in all phases, but SI significantly changed in the 3rd phase.

Thus, the major changes in the state of central hemodynamics in the rest of the lying were observed in the luteal phase of the OMC, which disappeared in various loads on the body (respiration 6 times/min, orthopedic, and psychoemotional load).

The cardiovascular system of the human body is one of the most important physiological systems, in the functioning of which involved rhythmic processes that interact with each other. The most important of these is the main cardiac rhythm and breathing.

When analyzing the parameters of the wave structure of the heart rate at rest, it was found that significant differences between their levels, depending on the phase of the OC, were largely absent. The exception is higher values of HFnorm in the III phase of the OC compared with II (65.4 [54.8, 75.0] and 55.4 [42.6, 68.9]%, respectively) and less aLF (11,533 [5449, 23,958] and 17,224 [9769, 26,508] ms^{2}*Hz-1, respectively), indicating a higher level of activation of the parasympathetic branch of the autonomic nervous system (VNS) in the follicular and luteal phases.

During orthogonal testing, there were significant changes in the wave structure of the cardiac rhythm that had certain features in different phases of the CMC. Thus, the level of VLF did not change, LF probably ($p < 0.05$) decreased from 670 [273, 974] to 459 [276, 689] ms^2 only in the 2nd phase. Significantly ($p < 0.001$) in all phases, HF, HFnorm, and TP decreased. Similar changes are the characteristic for this type of load and consist in increasing the tone of the sympathetic link of the CNS [17, 58, 59].

Under conditions of regulated breathing, minor changes in heart rhythm values were observed. Thus, the value of VLF changed in the second phase, and LF in the third phase is devastating with the I and II phases. The value of a LF showed significant changes in all phases (**Table 3**).

At a psychoemotional load, VLF did not change, LF was likely to decrease from 2.0 [1.1, 4.3] to 3.4 [1.8, 5.7] ms^2 only in the 2nd phase ($p < 0.05$). Significantly ($p < 0.001$) in all phases, HF and aLF increased.

The analysis of the cardiac rhythm reactivity in orthostatic conditions (**Table 4**) showed that in the luteal phase, an increase in the power of low frequency waves of heart rate was observed, which was significantly higher than the amplitude of their decrease in the ovulatory phase. Also, in the 3rd phase, there was a significant increase in the maximum peak in the frequency range of 0.04–0.15 Hz (60.8%).

In regulated breathing, the changes in all phases were in VLF, aLF, and TPover. Insignificant in HF and HFnorm (**Table 5**).

It is noteworthy that the greatest deviation of the values of reactivity to the load is typical for indicators that characterize the frequency range of oscillations R-R from 0.04 to 0.15 Hz.

Indicator	Phases of the cycle		
	I	II	III
VLF, мs²	9.33 [6.44; 12.49]	6.65 [3.48; 13.56]*	6.84 [3.47; 11.19]
LF, мs²	33.11 [13.48; 43.05]	38.36 [18.76; 57.03]*	42.09 [20.9; 59.79]#
HF, мс²	18.9 [10.9; 35.32]	20.9 [13.83; 33.71]*	21.98 [14.36; 33.05]
aLF, мs²/Гц	23.61 [8.53; 57.74]	39.19 [17.80; 63.68]*	32.28 [15.23; 83.52]#
HFnorm, %	40.82 [28.74; 52.61]	36.68 [26.36; 49.77]*	36.01 [23.04; 47.87]
TPover, мs²	62.87 [48.09; 98.42]	62.98 [46.90; 103.43]	70.24 [48.9; 103.33]#

*–$p < 0.05$ in comparison with indicators in phase I.
#–$p < 0.05$ in between the indices in the 2nd and 3rd phases.

Table 3. Indices of the variability of the heart rate at regulated respiration (6 times/min) in different phases of the biological cycle.

Indicator	Phases of the cycle		
	I	II	III
VLF	−15.8 [−49.5; 43.5]	−20.4 [−57.5; 25.8]	−8.9 [−46.3; 64.8]
LF	−1.4 [−35.6; 60.8]	−21.7 [−59.2; 29.7]	27.6# [−35; 71.8]
HF	−73.4 [−88.7; −3.5]	−70.8 [−85.5; −1.3]	−73.3 [−83.4; −5.2]
aLF	14.1 [−21.5; 127]	24 [−38.4; 88.3]	60.8# [−2.2; 228.6]
fLF	−8.5 [−45.8; 20.3]	−5.8 [−27.5; 14.7]	−19.6 [−38.4; 19.6]
HFnorm	−56.5 [−65.9; −39.2]	−50.8 [−60.6; −34.3]	−49.3 [−64.3; −40.9]
TP	−38.7 [−59.5; 0]	−41.3 [−71.2; 7.3]	−35.7 [−52.6; 32.5]

*−$p < 0.05$ in comparison with indicators in phase I.
#−$p < 0.05$ in between the indices in the 2nd and 3rd phases.

Table 4. Reactivity (%) of heart rate variability parameters at orthopedic examination in different phases of the biological cycle of women (median, borders 25, 75 percentiles).

Indicator	Phases of cycle		
	I	II	III
VLF, $мс^2$	74.4 [2.38; 147.47]	2.68 [−46.24; 98.00]*	−29.13 [−51.01; 29.53]#
LF, $мс^2$	33.1 [13.48; 43.05]	38.36 [18.76; 57.03]	42.09 [20.9; 59.59]#
HF, $мс^2$	19.0 [10.96; 35.32]	20.90 [13.83; 33.71]	21.98 [14.36; 33.03]
aLF, $мс^2$/Hz	1850 [905; 2949]	1966 [545; 3034]*	2195 [1070; 4148]#
HFnorm, %	−56.2 [−64.07; −28.71]	−52.44 [−67.53; −33.49]	−52.38 [−71.19; -40.89]
TPover, $мс^2$	77.6 [8.24; 220.25]	62.10 [6.06; 172.36]*	90.79 [46.71; 171.50]#

*−$p < 0.05$ in comparison with indicators in phase I.
#−$p < 0.05$ in between the indices in the 2nd and 3rd phases.

Table 5. Reactivity (%) of parameters of heart rate variability during regulated breathing (6 times/min) in different phases of the biological cycle of women (median, borders of 25 and 75 percentiles).

In this regard, a detailed analysis of the distribution of waves of the cardiac rhythm in it was performed on a normalized median spectrogram.

6. Discussion

As for the phases of the menstrual cycle, Princi from the sing did not find changes in the heart rate in three phases [47]. However, in our study, analyzing the heart rate reactivity, we found that in the luteal phase, an increase in the power of low frequency waves of heart rate was observed, which was significantly higher than the amplitude of their decrease in the ovulatory phase. Also, in the 3rd phase, there was a significant increase in the maximum peak in the frequency range of 0.04–0.15 Hz (60.8%).

According to Princi with singing, the total power of the spectrum and its high frequency part increased in the folliculin phase and decreased during the luteal phase.

Leicht et al. noted a high heart rate in the ovulation phase at a constant level of all endogenous hormones, and even the variability of the heart rate was the same in different phases of the cycle. However, they identified the correlation between the level of estrogen and the absolute expression of HRV in ovulation. The correlations found between the peak of estrogen and HRV are attributed to the cardioprotective effect of hormones in healthy women.

Tanaka et al. (2003) believe that the cardiovascular reflex may be damaged depending on the level of estradiol Guasti (1999) studying autonomic function in the normal ovulatory cycle and evaluating HRV sensitivity of baroreceptors in healthy women. They found increased sympathetic activity in the second phase of the cycle. This gave reason to speak of different baro-reflex sensitivity in different phases of the cycle.

Investigating the state of hemodynamics and HRV in the studied group of women in different conditions, it was found that the nature of the distribution of spectral power in different phases of the CMC is significantly different. At rest, the phase I is characterized by one peak at a frequency of 0.1 Hz, and for II and III phases, there are two peaks that can have different mechanisms of origin [47]. Moreover, in the third phase, the wave at frequency 0.08 Hz, which according to the experimental data characterize the functioning of the baroreflex [22], is most pronounced. These results largely coincide with the conclusions of many authors that HRV is a genetically determined characteristic of a human body [9].

Princi [47] indicate that cardiointerval analysis is more appropriate to determine the slight variations in the VNS activity during the menstrual cycle than the use of traditional indicators such as heart rate and arterial pressure. It should be noted that the phase of the ovarian cycle can significantly affect the HRV in women of reproductive age, both at rest and in psycho-emotional stress (features of the cardiovascular system in different phases of the menstrual cycle) [28]. In our study, we found that during the neurodynamic load, significant adaptive changes in vegetative regulation in the follicular phase were observed, while the lowest reactivity and inhibition of the functional state of the organism were characteristic of the luteal phase of the CMC. In this case, in the conditions of a 10-minute neurodynamic test in the feedback mode using the method MV Makarenko, the number of processed signals was significantly higher in phase I (1533 [1309, 1642] signal) compared with II and III ([1438 [1219, 1573] signal) phases ($p < 0.05$). We believe that such changes in mental performance are due to changes in the hormonal status in the body of women. We also found that in the first phase, the difference between the ratio of correct answers of the right (52 [50, 54]%) and the left (48 [46, 50]%) hands was highly reliable ($p < 0.01$), while in II and III phases was leveled ($p < 0.501$ and 0.223, respectively). Such a pattern indicates the possibility of changes in the degree of domination of the cerebral hemispheres during the menstrual cycle.

However, the study by Grossman et al. [45] found no differences in the parameters of the wave structure of arterial pressure and heart rate when performing orthopedic and stimulating carotid sinus in women in different phases of the CMC.

In a study by Lawrence et al., studies, for 10 completely healthy women, it was found that spontaneous baroreflectory sensitivity increases during the luteal phase compared to the follicular phase.

By analyzing the distribution of cardiac heart rate wavelengths by normalized median spectrogram, we found that normalized spectral power in the range of low heart rate rhythms at orthodontic tests in men and women significantly differed at frequencies of 0.08 and 0.1 Hz. The latter can testify to the sexual characteristics of spontaneous baro-reflex sensitivity, a certain difference in the genesis of these waves.

The presence of two peaks can indicate two impacts on the heart rate spectrograph. Yes, there are two theories of wave formation in the low frequency region. The first is the effect of the functioning of the baroreflector mechanism of regulation of arterial pressure [60], and the second is the influence of the endogenous rhythm generator. In studies by Cooley et al. [27] evaluated the spectra of fluctuations in blood pressure and RR intervals in patients with implanted artificial left ventricle. After a short time after implantation (1 and 15 months), there were no slow waves in the arterial pressure spectra, and in the spectra of RR-intervals of their own heart, slow fluctuations "became apparent and dominant." The endogenous oscillator is likely to capture the rhythm of waves caused by the activity of the baro-reflex mechanism, which is a manifestation of the fundamental natural synchronization phenomenon [61], and in this case, the frequency of both the baroreflex and the oscillator is the same or slightly different.

A probable increase in the level of blood pressure in the 3rd phase compared with the 2nd and even the greater is the phase I, indicating an increase in the tone of the sympathetic department of the autonomic nervous system and is consistent with the literature data (Princi et al., 2005). Some authors [52] point out the individual peculiarities of autonomic regulation in women and predict the relative stability of the type of autonomous regulation and its genetic determinism. However, there are certain contradictions. Thus, Japanese scientists [43] observed an increase in the value of LF, which reflects the effect of both the sympathetic and parasympathetic VSS on the level of AT in both I and II phases.

But Princi and sang. (Princi et al., 2005) found opposite data, that is, the growth of LF in phase I and its decline in III. But only six women were screened and therefore, in our opinion, data for statistical processing are not enough. Lucini and sang (Lucini et al., [6]) noted an increase in blood pressure in the 2nd phase. In this case, the content of sex hormones did not change. It is also noted that the HRV indices did not change in any phase of CMC. However, a correlation between the content of estrogen and the absolute peak of HRV in the 2nd phase was identified. The found correlation is attributed to the cardiotropic effect of sex hormones. The autonomic nervous system plays a significant role in the processes of adaptation of the organism, and resulting in its functional state is very variable. Dependence of types of hemodynamics from the initial vegetative tone is considered in some diseases of the cardiovascular system. Establishing this relationship in the norm allows us to clarify algorithms for diagnosing the adaptive capacity of the organism, since they depend not only on the initial level of functioning of the system and functional reserves, which are most often used in medical-pedagogical control and preventive medicine, but also from the level of voltage regulatory systems, which is practically not taken into account.

In our study, we measured the level of vegetative tone with the HFnorm. Analysis of the distribution of this indicator in the first phase of CMC allowed to distinguish three typological groups: sympatotonic with a level up to 44% (19 people), norm tonics within the range of 44–60%, and vagogonics from 60% (26 people).

Probable differences in blood pressure levels between individuals of these typological groups were mainly found by diastolic blood pressure. So at rest, lying in the first phase of the CMC in BT, this indicator was higher than that of CT. At orthogonal testing of ATD in the 3rd phase of OMC in NT and VH was higher than in CT. Such shifts in values are also confirmed by the analysis of the reactivity of this indicator in the transition to orthostatic position. In BT, it is probably lower than CT in the first phase of CMC. While in the third phase of CMC in ST, there was no probable increase in comparison with the level of resting lying, and then in VT, this increase was not natural.

Thus, experimental studies have shown that an integrated approach to the study of individual-typological characteristics of central hemodynamics and its wave manifestations in women in different phases of the CMC gives an opportunity to answer a number of questions that arise in this case.

Based on the results of the study, we formulated the following conclusions:

1. Theoretical analysis of scientific and methodological literature has shown that there are certain contradictions in the results of various studies of the variability of the heart rate in women in different phases of the ovarian-menstrual cycle and the interpretation of their mechanisms, individually its changes to different loads.

2. In a state of rest in women, there are changes in the levels of systolic blood pressure and blood pressure in the central luteal phase of the OC compared with the follicular and ovulatory phases. The analysis of cardiac rhythm reactivity during ortho-trial in the luteal phase was characterized by an increase in the power of low frequency waves of heart rate, as well as a significant increase in the maximum peak in the frequency range of 0.04–0.15 Hz (60.8%).

3. Lying alone, with orthogonal and psychoemotional stress, there are basically differences in the parameters of the vibration duration of the interval R-R and UOC and their synchronization in women in ovulatory and luteinous phases compared to follicle. There is a significant link between Mayer's wave power and median and diastolic pressure, mainly in the women's follicular phase of CMC in all conditions. The maximum peak amplitude of the UOC spectrograph in the range of 0.04–0.15 Hz is most closely related to the levels of APm and APd.

Author details

Olena Lutsenko

Address all correspondence to: olena85lutsenko@gmail.com

Department of Theory and Methods of Teaching of Natural Sciences, Hlukhiv National Pedagogical University of Alexander Dovzhenko, Hlukhiv, Ukraine

References

[1] Angela R, Gregg P, Pierson A. Ovarian antral folliculogenesis during the human menstrual cycle. Human Reproduction Update. 2012;**18**(1):73-91

[2] Brooks VL, Cassaglia PA, Goldman RK. Baroreflex function in females: Changes with the reproductive cycle and pregnancy. Gender Medicine. 2012;**9**:61-67

[3] MacNaughton J, Banah M, McCloud P. Age related changes in follicle stimulating hormone, luteinizing hormone, oestradiol and immunoreactive inhibin in women of reproductive age. Clinical Endocrinology. 2008;**36**:339-345

[4] Glushkovskaya-Semyachkina OV, Anishchenko TG. Normalized entropy applied to the study of sex differences in cardiolovascular response to atropine and propranolol in normal and stressed rats. Computers in Cardiology. 2001;**28**:469-472

[5] Green JH. Cardiac vagal efferent activity in the cat. The American Journal of Physiology. 1959;**149**(1):47-49

[6] Lucini D, Norbiato G, Clerici M. Hemodynamic and autonomic adjustments to real life stress conditions in humans. Hypertension. 2002;**39**:184-188

[7] Aubert AE, Seps B, Beckers F. Heart rate variability in athletes. Sports Medicine. 2003; **33**(12):889-919

[8] Brown SJ. The effect a respiratory acidosis on human heart rate variability. Advances in Experimental Medicine and Biology. 2008;**605**:361-365

[9] Mohrman DE, Heller LJ. Cardiovascular Physiology. McGraw-Hill: Lange Medical Books; 2002. p. 257

[10] Lutsenko OI, Kovalenko SO. Blood pressure and hemodynamics: Mayer waves in different phases of ovarian and menstrual cycle in women. Physiological Research. 2017;**66**:235-240

[11] Karemaker JM. Analysis of blood pressure and heart rate variability: Theoretical consideration and clinical applicability. In: Clinical autonomic disorders. Evaluation and management. Boston: Little, Broun; 1993. pp. 315-330

[12] Pokrovskii VM. Alternative viev on the mechanism of cardiac rhythmogenesis. Heart, Lung & Circulation. 2003;**12**:18-24

[13] Kontosic I, Mesaros-Kanjski E, Bozin-Juracic J. Some anthropometric characteristics, reactions on physical stress, and blood pressure in males aged 18 in «Primorsko-Goranska» County. Collegium Antropologicum. 2001;**1**:31-39

[14] Karavaev AS, Ponomarenko VI. Synchronization of low-frequency oscillations in the human cardiovascular system. Chaos. 2009;**19**:33-112

[15] Kovalenko SO, Kudij LI, Lutsenko OI. Peculiarities of male and female heart rate variability. Science and Education a New Dimension. 2013;**1(2)**(15):17-20

[16] Lucy SD, Hughson RL, Kowalchuk JM. Body position and cardiac dynamic and chronotropic responses to steadystate isocapnic hypoxaemia in humans. Experimental Physiology. 2000;**85**:227-237

[17] Montano N, Gnecchi Ruscone T, Porta A. Presence of vasomotor and respiratory rhythms in the discharge of single medullary neurons involved in the regulation of cardiovascular system. Journal of the Autonomic Nervous System. 1996;**57**:116-122

[18] Rilling JK. A potential role for oxytocin in the intergenerational transmission of secure attachment. Neuropsychopharmacology. 2009;**34**(13):2621-2622

[19] Cella F, Giordano G, Cordera R. Serum leptin concentrations during the menstrual cycle in normal-weight women: Effects of an oral triphasic estrogen-progestin medication. European Journal of Endocrinology. 2000;**142**:174

[20] Donovan T, Bosch SS. Physiology of Puberty. London: Edward Arnold Ltd.; 1965

[21] Lewandowski J. Sex hormone modulation of neuropeptide Y and cardiovascular responses to stress in humans. In: Stress: Molecular Genetic and Neurobiological Advances. Gordon and Breach Science Publishers S.A., New York, USA; 1996. pp. 569-578

[22] Nakagawa M. Influence of menstrual cycle on QT interval dynamics. Pacing and Clinical Electrophysiology. 2006:607-613

[23] Purdon SE. Menstrual effects on asymmetrical olfactory acuity. Journal of the International Neuropsychological Society. 2001;**6**:703-709

[24] Siepka SM, Yoo SH, Lee C. Genetics and neurobiology of circadian clocks in mammals. Cold Spring Harbor Symposia on Quantitative Biology. 2007;**72**:251-259

[25] Collins P. Vascular aspects of oestrogen. Journal of the Climacteric and Postmenopause. 1996;**23**:217-226

[26] Cooke WN. Head rotation during upright tilt increases cardiovagal baroreflex sensitivity. Aviation, Space, and Environmental Medicine. 2007;**5**:463-469

[27] Cooley RL, Montano N, Cogliati C. Evidence for a central origin of the low-frequency oscillation in RR-interval variability. Circulation. 1998;**98**(6):556-561

[28] Johansson T, Ritzen EM. Very long-term follow-up of girls with early and late menarche. Endocrine Development. 2005;**8**:26-36

[29] Malhotra A. Effects of sex hormones on development of physiological and pathological hypertrophy in male and female rats. The American Journal of Physiology. 1990; **259**:866-871

[30] Manzo A, Ootaki Y, Ootaki C. Comparative study of heart rate variability between healthy human subjects and healthy dogs, rabbits and calves. Laboratory Animals. 2009; **43**:41-45

[31] Fluckiger L. Differential effects of aging on heart rate variability and blood pressure variability. Journal of Gerontology: Biological Sciences. 1999;**5**:219-224

[32] Anishchenko TG, Glushkovskaya-Semyachkina OV. Normalized entropy applied to the analysis of gender-related differences in parasympathetic cardiovascular control in normal and stressed rat. Physician and Technology. 2003;**34**(1):29-39

[33] Gevese A, Gulli G, Polati E. Baroreflex and oscillation of heart period at 0.1 Hz studied by a-blokade and cross-spectral analysis of healthy humans. The Journal of Physiology. 2001;**1**:235-244

[34] Gipson IK, Moccia R, Spurr-Michaud S. The amount of MUC5B mucin in cervical mucus peaks at midcycle. Clinics in Endocrinology and Metabolism. 2001;**86**:594-595

[35] Girdler SS. Hemodynamic stress responses in men and womenexamined as a function of female menstrual cycle phase. International Journal of Psychophysiology. 1994; **17**(3):233-248

[36] Glass L. Introduction to controversial topics in nonlinear science: Is the normal heart rate chaotic. Chaos. 2009;**19**:28-50

[37] Hirshoren N. Menstrual cycle effects on the neurohumoral and autonomic nervous systems regulating the cardiovascular system. Clinics in Endocrinology and Metabolism. 2002;**4**:1569-1575

[38] Sanders G, Sjodin M, de Chastelaine M. On the elusive nature of sex differences in cognition: Hormonal influences contributing to within-sex variation. Archives of Sexual Behavior. 2002;**1**:145-152

[39] Sato N, Miyake S. Cardiovascular reactivity to mental stress: Relationship with menstrual cycle and gender. Journal of Physiological Anthropology and Applied Human Science. 2004;**23**:215-223

[40] Sayers BM. Analysis of heart rate variability. Ergonomics. 1973;**16**:17-32

[41] Scheer FL, Hiltona M, Mantzoros CS. Adverse metabolic and cardiovascular consequences of circadian misalignment. Proceedings of the National Academy of Sciences of the United States of America. 2009;**106**:4453-4458

[42] Schüring AN, Busch AS, Bogdanova N. Effects of the FSH-β-subunit promoter polymorphism -211G->T on the hypothalamic-pituitary-ovarian axis in normally cycling women indicate a gender-specific regulation of gonadotropin secretion. Clinics in Endocrinology and Metabolism. 2013;**98**:82-86

[43] Yamamoto M, Tsutsumi Y, Furukawa K. Influence of normal menstrual cycle on autonomic nervous activity and QT Dispersion. International Journal of Bioelectromagnetism. 2003:152-153

[44] Koenig JI, Jarczok MN, Ellis RJ. Body mass index is related to autonomic nervous system activity as measured by heart rate variability. Clinical Nutrition. 2009;**63**(10):1263-1265

[45] Grossman P, Taylor EW. Toward understanding respiratory sinus arrhythmia: Relations to cardiac vagal tone, evolution and biobehavioral functions. Biological Psychology. 2007;**74**(2):263-285

[46] Holzen JJ. Impact of endo- and exogenous estrogens on heart rate variability in women: A review. Climacteric. 2016;**1**:222-228

[47] Princi TS. Parametric evaluation of heart rate variability during the menstrual cycle in young women. Biomedical Sciences Instrumentation. 2005:340-345

[48] Taylor AE, Whitney H, Hall JE. Midcycle levels of sex steroids are sufficient to recreate the follicle-stimulating hormone but not the luteinizing hormone midcycle surge: Evidence for the contribution of other ovarian factors to the surge in normal women. Clinics in Endocrinology and Metabolism. 1995;**80**:15-41

[49] Tenan MS, Brothers RM, Tweedell AJ. Changes in resting heart rate variability across the menstrual cycle. Psychophysiology. 2014;**51**(10):996-1004

[50] Celeste NT, Mickiewicz AL. The role of the ventral pallidum in psychiatric disorders psychiatric disorders. Neuropsychopharmacology. 2010;**35**(1):337

[51] Vallais F, Baselli G, Lucini D. Spontaneous baroreflex sensitivity estimates during graded bicycle exercise: A comparative study. Physiological Measurement. 2009;**30**:201

[52] Welt CK, McNicholl DJ, Taylor AE, Hall JE. Female reproductive aging is marked by decreased secretion of dimeric inhibin. Clinics in Endocrinology and Metabolism. 1999;**84**:105

[53] Kuczmierczyk AR. Autonomic arousal and pain sensitivity in women with premenstrual syndrome at different phases of the menstrual cycle. Journal of Psychosomatic Research. 1986;**30**(4):421-428

[54] Makarenko MV. Method of conducting surveys and evaluation of individual neurodynamic properties of human higher nervous activity. Physiological Journal. 1999;**4**. t.45:125-131

[55] Kubichek WG. Impedanse cardiography as a noninvasive method of monitoring cardiac function and other parameters of the cardiovascular system. Annals of the New York Academy of Sciences. 1970;**2**:724-732

[56] A.S. Computer program for the registration and analysis of heart rate and respiration (CASPICO)/Kovalenko SO, Yakovlev ME. No. 11262; stated. 04.10.2004; has published Feb 15, 2005. Bul. No. 6

[57] Influence of tilt-test on a functional state of women cardiovascular system in the different phases of menstrual cycle Interdisciplinary. Scientific Conference «Adaptation Strategies of the Living Systems» 12-17 May 2012, AR Crimea; AR Crimea; 2012. pp. 22-23

[58] Fisher JP, Kim A, Hartwich D. New insights into the effects of age and sex on arterial baroreflex function at rest and during dynamic exercise in humans. Autonomic Neuroscience. 2012;**172**:13-22

[59] Muscelli E, Emdin M, Natali A. Autonomic and hemodynamic responses to insulin in lean and obese humans. Clinics in Endocrinology and Metabolism. 1998;**6**:2084-2090

[60] Chapuis B, Vidal-Petiot E, Oréa V. Linear modelling analysis of baroreflex control of arterial pressure variability in rats. The Journal of Physiology. 2004;**559**:639-649

[61] Baker FC. Circadian rhythms, sleep and the menstrual cycle. Sleep Medicine. 2007; **8**(6):613-622

Chapter 3

Influence of Branching Patterns and Active Contractions of the Villous Tree on Fetal and Maternal Blood Circulations in the Human Placenta

Yoko Kato

Additional information is available at the end of the chapter

http://dx.doi.org/10.5772/intechopen.79343

Abstract

In the human placenta, fetal blood circulates in the blood vessels of the villous tree while maternal one circulates in the intervillous space, the surroundings of the villous tree. Previously, the computational model of the villous tree, whose stem villi actively contract because of the contractile cells, has been developed. The result of the computation indicated that the displacement caused by the contraction would be helpful for the fetal and maternal circulations and can be combined with the other measurements for blood circulations in the placenta. Hypoxia in the placenta is classified into the following categories: preplacental hypoxia, uteroplacental hypoxia, and postplacental hypoxia. The number and the form of the terminal villi are altered by hypoxia. Assuming that increase in the terminal villi causes a higher shear elastic modulus of the placenta, this villous tree model is useful to estimate the influence of hypoxia on the blood circulations. In this chapter, how these three types of hypoxia influence the blood circulation in the placenta by the aforementioned computational model are discussed. While preplacental hypoxia and uteroplacental hypoxia would cause similar displacement in large regions, postplacental hypoxia would do vice versa. All the types might make the fetal and maternal blood circulations difficult.

Keywords: placenta, hypoxia, villous tree, terminal villi, contraction, blood circulation

1. Introduction

In the human placenta, the blood vessels in the villous tree lead to the umbilical artery and vein, while the intervillous space, the surroundings of the villous tree, is linked to the uterine artery

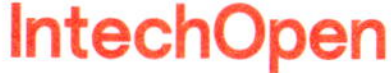

and vein. The fetal and maternal blood circulates separately so that the substances and gases are exchanged through the surface of the villous tree, without mixing these two types of blood [1]. The influence of the blood circulations on the exchange of the substances has been investigated [2, 3]. Also, the fetal and maternal blood circulations in the placenta have been evaluated by ultrasound Doppler and MRI so that the influences of these circulations on fetal growth have been indicated [4–9]. However, the direction of the blood flow in the placenta has been hardly determined yet.

The villous tree is classified into the following villous types: stem villi, intermediate villi, terminal villi, and mesenchymal villi [1, 10]. At term, the villous tree is mainly composed of stem villi, mature intermediate villi, and terminal villi [1, 11, 12]. The stem villi, the main support of the villous tree, are connected to the mature intermediate villi, which is accompanied by the terminal villi. In the stem villi, arteries, veins, arterioles, venules, and capillaries are observed [1, 11]. The mature intermediate villi have arteriole, postcapillary venules, and capillaries, part of which are linked to the capillary loop in the terminal villi [1, 12]. The artery and vein in the stem villi are surrounded by contractile cells, which are axially aligned [13–20]. Also, the contraction of the stem villi has been observed [14, 21–23].

Since the contraction of the stem villi would contribute to the fetal and maternal blood circulations in the placenta, the computational model of the villous tree, which actively contracts, has been developed [24]. In this model, the contraction of the stem villi causes the displacement of the surroundings: the displacement propagates from the surface of the stem villi. The result of the computation based on this model indicated that the magnitude of the displacement was almost kept in the placenta, and the direction was helpful for the fetal and maternal circulations although several positions were vulnerable to the mechanical properties of the placenta [24]. In addition, the comparison between the displacement pattern estimated by this model and flow velocity measured by the aforementioned methods will provide the direction of the blood flow in the placenta [24]. However, how the parameters in this computation, including the shear elastic modulus of the placenta and the maximum distance for the propagation, influence the displacement has not been investigated yet.

Hypoxia is classified into the following groups: preplacental hypoxia, less oxygen content in the maternal blood; uteroplacental hypoxia, normal oxygen content in the maternal blood but less content in the uteroplacental tissues; postplacental hypoxia, normal oxygen content in the maternal blood but less content in the fetus because of the problem in the fetoplacental perfusion [1, 25, 26]. In preplacental hypoxia and uteroplacental hypoxia, capillaries are highly branched and the terminal villi are clustered so that the terminal villi are predominantly observed [1, 25, 26]. The terminal villi in postplacental hypoxia are filiform and scarcely observed [1, 25, 26]. The villous tree model, which changes its shape based on the oxygen content, has also developed [27]. Assuming that an increase in the terminal villi is corresponding to the higher shear elastic modulus of the placenta and longer propagation distance of the stem villi contraction, the stem villi model [24] is useful to estimate the influence of hypoxia on the blood circulation in the placenta. However, such an analysis has not been done yet.

In this chapter, how three kinds of hypoxia influence the blood circulations in the placenta was evaluated. The computational model of the stem villi has been developed and used to estimate the distribution of the displacement in the placenta previously [24]. The distribution of the displacement was analyzed not for hypoxia, but for general characteristics of the displacement so that the influences of the parameters such as the shear elastic modulus and distance for the propagation on the displacement have barely investigated. After introducing the model of the villous tree, the analyses for the influences of these parameters on the displacement and characteristics of the displacement in hypoxia were indicated.

2. Computational models

2.1. Villous tree model

The computational model and parameters have been reported previously [24]. **Figure 1** shows the computational model, where the chorionic and basal plates are the boundaries for the fetal and maternal sites, respectively. Truncus chorii, rami chorii, and ramuli chorii are parts of the stem villi. The position in the model is indicated by the Cartesian coordinate: the z axis, whose origin is placed on the chorionic plate, perpendicular to the chorionic and basal plates. That is, the z coordinate is corresponding to the distance from the chorionic plate. The surroundings of the stem villi are composed of the intervillous space, where the maternal blood circulates, and all the villi except the stem villi. The size and branching patterns based on the histological reports [1, 10] were as follows: diameter, 3–0.3 mm; branching pattern, no bifurcation in the truncus chorii, equally dichotomous as well as symmetric in the rami chorii, and unequally dichotomous as well as asymmetric in the ramuli chorii.

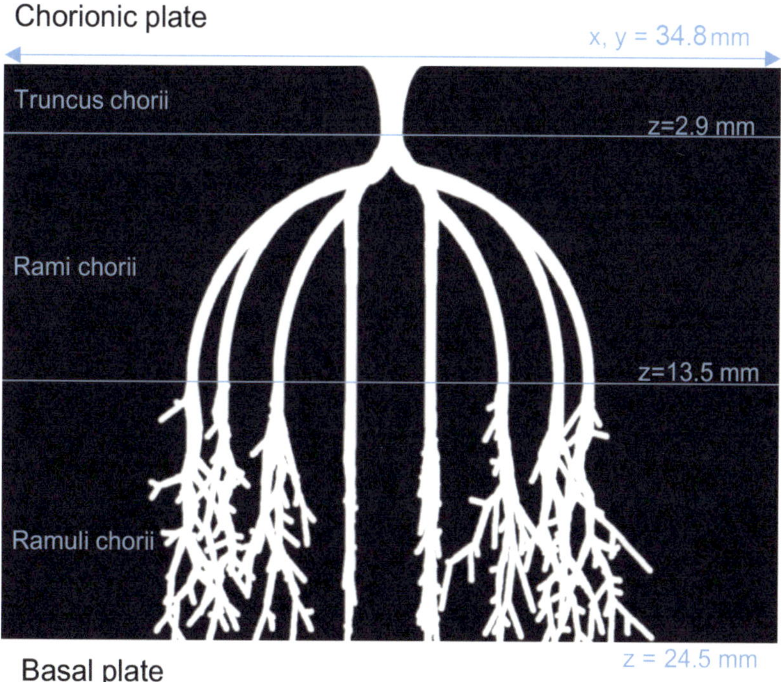

Figure 1. Side view of the villous tree model. White region, stem villi; black region, other types of villi and intervillous space; size (x, y, z), 1200 × 1200 × 847 pixels (1 pixel = 29 μm) (source: modified from Figure 1 in Kato et al. [24]).

The displacement, u, is described by the following equation:

$$u = \xi_o \cos kr \quad (1)$$

where ξ_o is the amplitude (0.1 μm), k is the wavenumber and r is the distance from the surface of the stem villi. The maximum distance for the propagation, s, was 1.45, 2.9, or 4.35 mm. Also, the shear elastic modulus, μ, is described as follows:

$$\mu = \rho \lambda^2 \upsilon^2 \quad (2)$$

where ϱ is the density (1.0×10^3 kg/m^3), λ is the wavelength (0.29, 0.58, or 1.45 mm), and ν is the frequency (1 Hz). Hence, the shear elastic modulus of the placenta was 8.41×10^{-5} Pa, 3.36×10^{-4} Pa, or 2.10×10^{-3} Pa. The displacement caused by the contraction was indicated by the polar coordinate: magnitude, ϕ (0 to 180°) and θ (−180 to 180°).

2.2. Hypoxia model

The villous tree in preplacental hypoxia and uteroplacental hypoxia has plenty of terminal villi while that in postplacental hypoxia has few filiform ones [1, 25, 26]. It was assumed that an increase in the number of the terminal villi makes the shear elastic modulus of the placenta higher and the maximum distance for the propagation of the displacement longer. Because the model, whose shear elastic modulus was 3.36×10^{-4} Pa, was the control model, the shear elastic moduli in the preplacental hypoxia and uteroplacental hypoxia model and the postplacental hypoxia model were 2.10×10^{-3} and 8.41×10^{-5} Pa, respectively. Also, the maximum distances for the displacement propagation of the preplacental hypoxia and uteroplacental hypoxia model and the postplacental model were 4.35 and 1.45 mm, respectively, since that of the control model was 2.9 mm. Because the shear elastic moduli and the maximum distance for the propagation had three types, respectively, nine different models were made. The models except the control model, the preplacental hypoxia and uteroplacental hypoxia model, and the postplacental model represent the conditions toward these types of hypoxia.

2.3. Contraction

Three types of hypoxia in the placenta alter the terminal villi but rarely the stem villi. How the hypoxia influences the contractile cells in the stem villi has been barely investigated. The previous report has indicated that fetal growth restriction enhances α-smooth muscle actin of the stem villi [28]. Hence, the amplitude, ξ_o, in Eq. (1) could be maintained in all the models but also be changed as 0.4 μm for 8.41×10^{-5} Pa, 0.016 μm for 2.10×10^{-3} Pa because of the change in the elastic moduli.

2.4. Characteristic positions

In order to evaluate the influence of the terminal villi on the displacement distribution in the placenta, the mean and standard deviation of the magnitude, ϕ and θ in each z coordinate were used as the previous report indicated [24]. The middle positions of each part and several z coordinates which show the characteristic distributions of the magnitude, ϕ, and θ are used: z_t, z_r, and z_{rl}, the middle positions of the truncus chorii, rami chorii, and ramuli chorii; $z_{sd/mean}$, the z coordinate at the peak of the standard deviation normalized by the mean in the displaced area; $z_{\phi 1}$ and $z_{\phi 2}$, the z coordinates at the lower and higher peaks of the standard deviation of ϕ, respectively; z_{θ}, the z coordinate at the lower peak of the mean from the rami chorii to the ramuli chorii. These positions have been used previously [24], but how the parameters influence the positions have not been investigated yet.

2.5. Statistical analysis

The coefficient of determination, R^2, in the regression line, and the number of the samples, n, provide F-value, F, whose $df1$ and $df2$ were 1 and $n-2$, respectively:

$$F = n-2\frac{R^2}{1-R^2} \tag{3}$$

The level of significance was 0.05.

3. Results

3.1. Displaced region

Figure 2 shows that the displaced volume normalized by the volume of the entire model except the stem villi region became larger as the maximum distance for the propagation, s, grew longer. However, the wavelength scarcely altered the size of the displaced region.

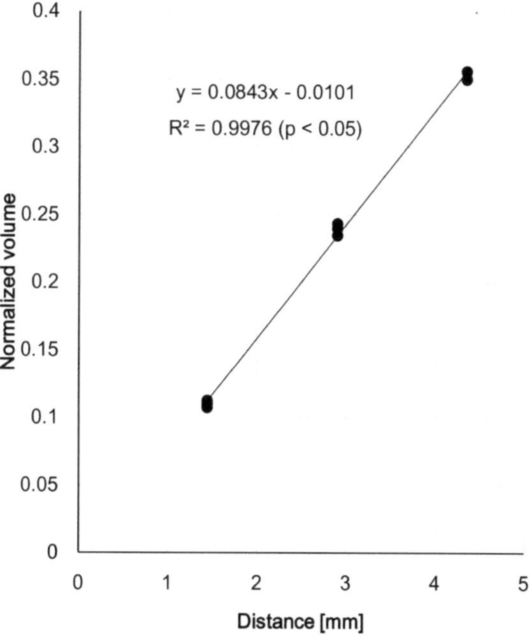

Figure 2. Displaced volume normalized by the volume of the model except the stem villi (2.96×10^4 mm^3).

These results indicate that the displaced area in the placenta under preplacental hypoxia and uteroplacental hypoxia would be larger than that under postplacental hypoxia.

Figure 3 shows the displaced area at the control model. Since the wavelength weakly influences the size of the displaced region, the mean of the displaced area at the same maximum distance for the propagation in each characteristic z coordinate was calculated. **Figure 4** show the relationship between the displaced area normalized by that at the maximum distance for the propagation of the control model (2.9 mm) and the characteristic z coordinates. The maximum distance for the propagation almost equally altered the size of the displaced area at all the characteristic position except z_t and $z_{sd/mean}$ at both of the maximum distances. The influence of the maximum distance on the size of the displaced area at z_t and $z_{sd/mean}$ were much larger than that on the other positions. Considering that z_t and $z_{sd/mean}$ are close to the chorionic plate, all the types of hypoxia would strongly influence the blood circulations near the chorionic plate.

3.2. Characteristic positions

Figure 5 shows that the maximum distance for the propagation scarcely influenced the characteristic z positions. The influence of the wavelength was also little. Hence, the characteristic z positions would be kept in all the types of hypoxia.

3.3. Displacement: magnitude

Figures 6 and **7** show the mean of the displacement in each model when the amplitude ξ_o was maintained. As the wavelength and maximum distance for the propagation grew

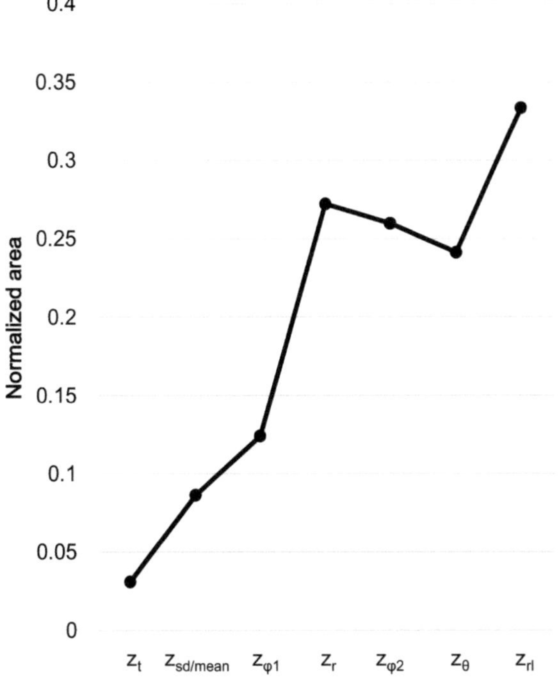

Figure 3. Displaced area normalized by the area of the model at each z coordinate. λ = 0.58 mm and s = 2.9 mm.

http://dx.doi.org/10.5772/intechopen.79343

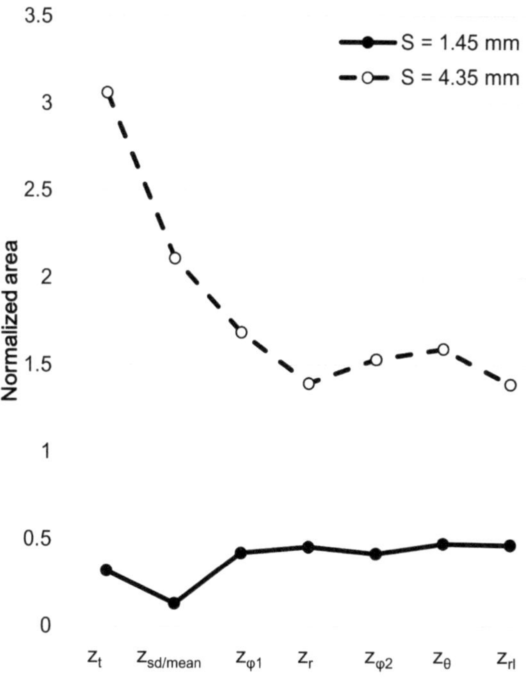

Figure 4. Displaced area normalized by that of the model for s = 2.9 mm at the characteristic z coordinates. The displaced area in each model (s = 1.45, 2.9, and 4.35 mm) was averaged.

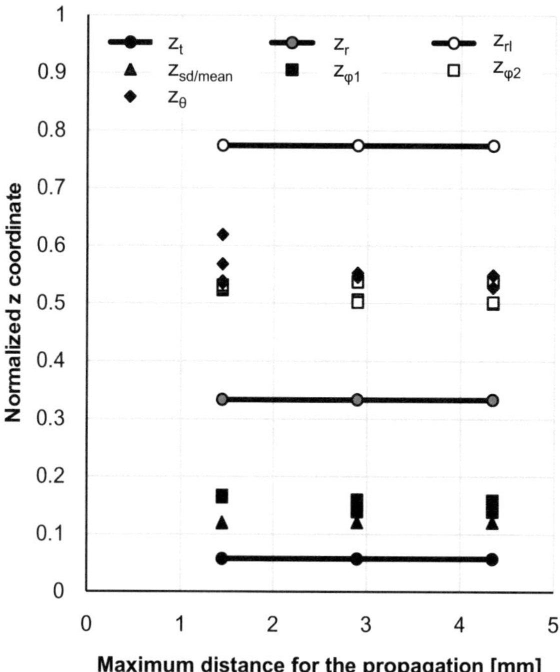

Figure 5. Distance from the characteristic positions to the chorionic plate normalized by that between the chorionic and basal plates.

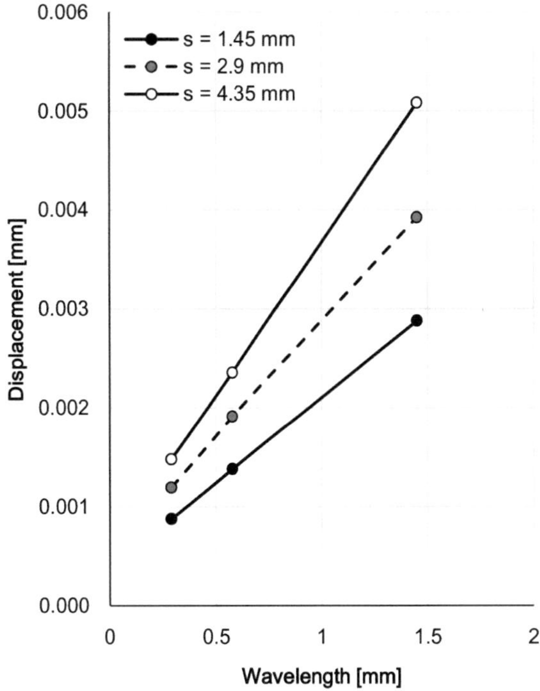

Figure 6. Influence of the wavelength on the mean of the displacement in each model.

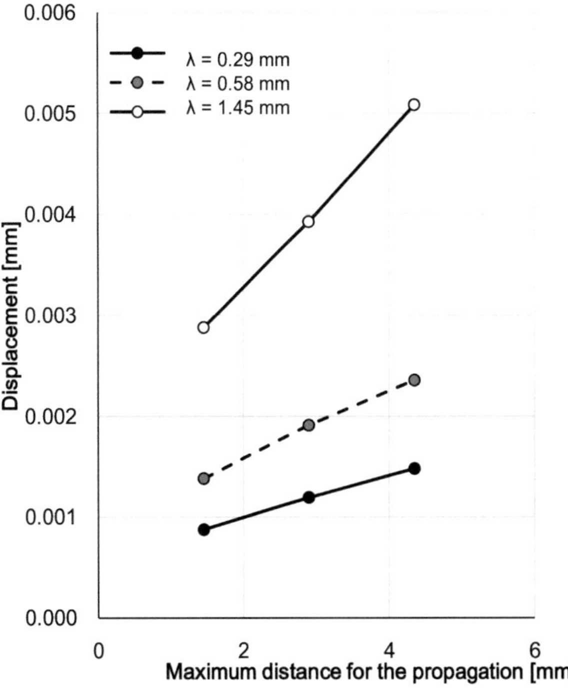

Figure 7. Influence of the maximum distance for the propagation on the mean of the displacement in each model.

longer, the displacement became larger. When ξ_o became smaller as the shear elastic modulus of the placenta grew larger, the mean of the displacement was largely decreased by the longer wavelength as **Figure 8** shows. In **Figure 9**, the longer distance for the propagation induced the larger displacement as shown in **Figure 7**. However, the longer wavelength induced the larger displacement in **Figure 7** but vice versa in **Figure 9**. Considering that the preplacental hypoxia and uteroplacental hypoxia model, and the postplacental hypoxia model showed the smallest elastic moduli and maximum distance, and the largest ones, the mean of the displacement would be different from the control model as shown in **Figures 6–9**.

3.4. Displacement: direction (ϕ and θ)

While **Figure 10** shows that the influence of the wavelength on the range of the area fraction for ϕ = 45–135° among those at the characteristic z coordinates was barely consistent, the longer maximum distance for the propagation reduced the range as shown in **Figure 11**. Hence, the longer maximum distance for the propagation would weaken the influence of the z coordinate on ϕ.

Both the wavelength and the maximum distance for the propagation influenced the standard deviation of the area fraction in each class interval of θ (SDin), but not consistently. SDin at z_r was decreased by the longer wavelength and maximum distance as shown in **Figure 12**. SDin at z_{rl} indicated the same tendency, but those at z_t and z_θ did not.

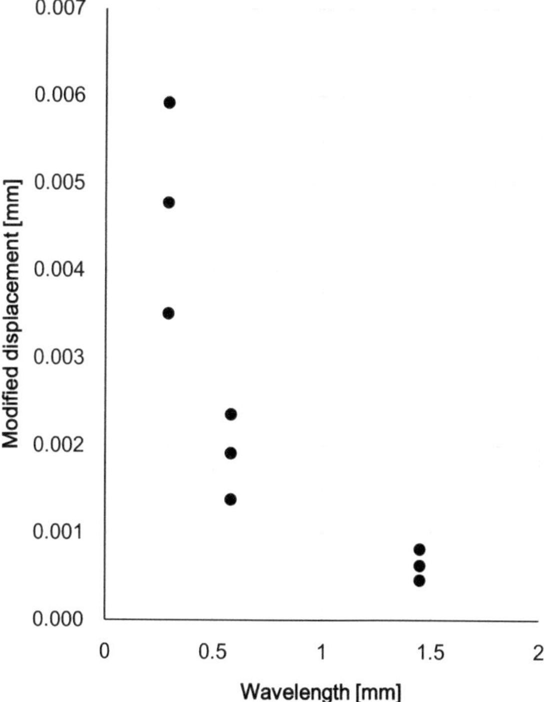

Figure 8. Influence of the wavelength on the mean of the modified displacement.

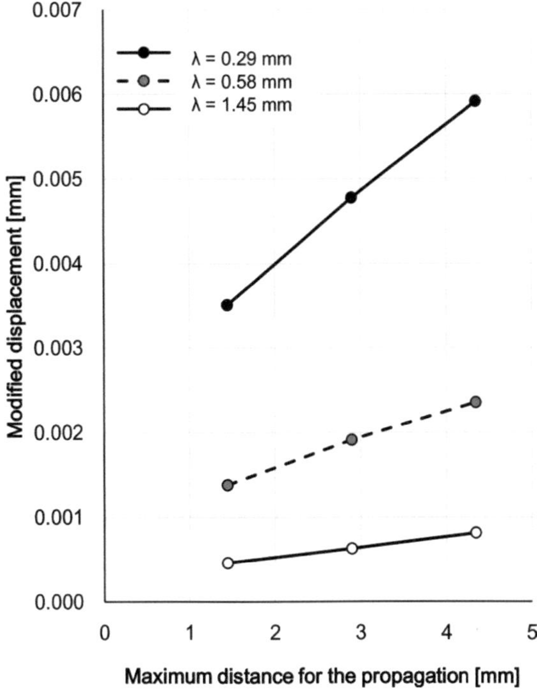

Figure 9. Influence of the maximum distance for the propagation on the mean of the modified displacement.

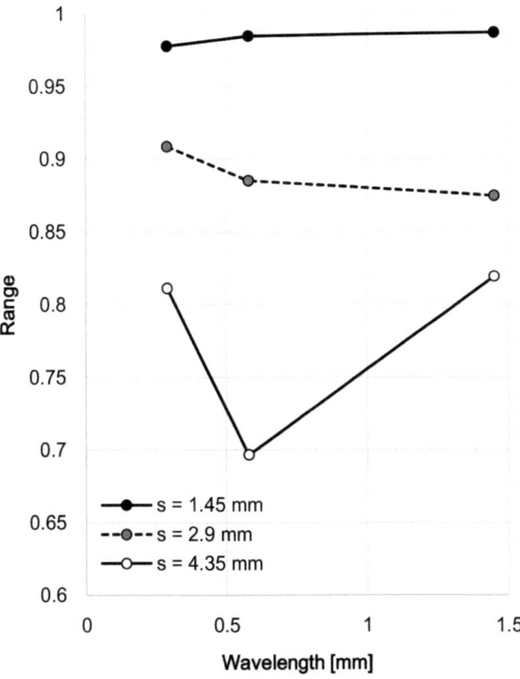

Figure 10. Influence of the wavelength on the range of the area fraction for the displaced area at $\phi = 45–135°$.

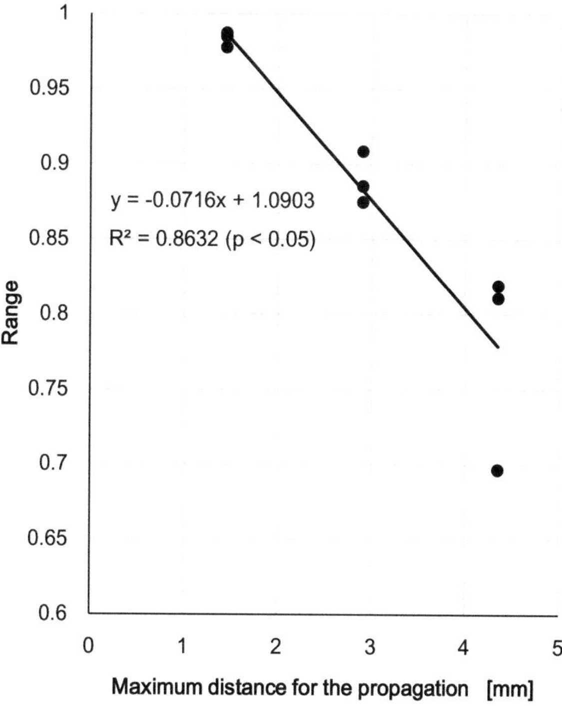

Figure 11. Influence of the Maximum distance for the propagation on the range of the area fraction for the displaced area at $\phi = 45–135°$.

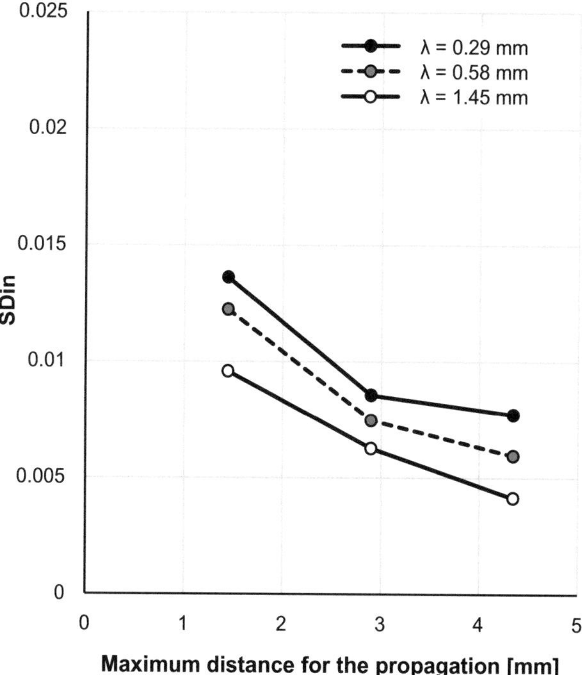

Figure 12. The standard deviation of the area fraction in each class interval of θ (SDin) at the rami chorii.

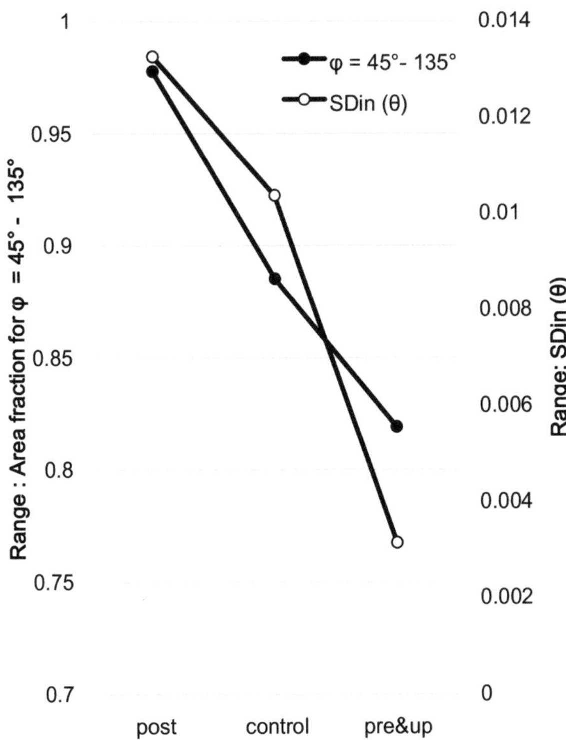

Figure 13. The range of the area fraction for 45–135°, and range of SDin (θ). Post, postplacental hypoxia; pre&up, preplacental hypoxia and uteroplacental hypoxia.

Figure 13 shows the ranges of the area fraction for ϕ = 45–135° and SDin at the control model (s = 2.9 mm, $\mu = 3.36 \times 10^{-4}$ Pa), postplacental hypoxia model (s = 1.45 mm, $\mu = 8.41 \times 10^{-5}$ Pa), and preplacental hypoxia and uteroplacental hypoxia model (s = 4.35 mm, $\mu = 2.10\times 10^{-3}$ Pa). In both ranges, the postplacental hypoxia model was the largest while the preplacental and uteroplacental hypoxia model was the smallest. The result described that the direction of the displacement in the postplacental hypoxia model was more varied than that in the preplacental hypoxia and uteroplacental hypoxia model.

4. Discussion

In this chapter, the displacement caused by the contraction of the stem villi in the three types of hypoxia in the placenta was evaluated. While the villous tree is rich in terminal villi at preplacental hypoxia and uteroplacental hypoxia, it has few terminal villi at postplacental hypoxia. Assuming that increase in the terminal villi in the placenta induces higher shear elastic moduli of the placenta, postplacental hypoxia would show lower shear elastic moduli while preplacental hypoxia and uteroplacental hypoxia would show higher ones. In the meantime, the computational model of the villous tree with active contractions has been developed previously [24], and it has been shown that the magnitude and direction of the displacement would be helpful for the blood circulation in the placenta [24]. Because the general aspects of the displacement caused by the contraction were investigated in the previous study [24], the influence of each parameter on the displacement and how to modulate the parameter and model for representing the dysfunction of the placenta, including hypoxia, has been barely discussed. Based on the previous computation [24], the analysis for the preplacental hypoxia and uteroplacental hypoxia model and the postplacental hypoxia model was done.

The maximum propagation distance influenced the displaced region, especially near the chorionic plate. However, the characteristic z coordinates, was not influenced by the shear elastic modulus and the maximum propagation distance. When increase in the shear elastic modulus of the placenta reduced the displacement caused by the contraction of the stem villi, the placenta in preplacental hypoxia or uteroplacental hypoxia caused smaller displacement than that in postplacental hypoxia. Also, changes in the magnitude and direction of the displacement would occur at the characteristic positions, kept in all the models. The range of the area fraction for the displaced area at $\phi = 45–135°$ got smaller as the maximum distance for the propagation became longer. The influence of the wavelength and the maximum distance for the propagation on the standard deviation of the area fraction in each class interval of θ (SDin) was dependent on the z coordinates. The SDin was more influenced by the z coordinates than the wavelength and the maximum distance so that SDin would be dependent on the shape of the stem villi. The ranges of the area fraction at $\phi = 45–135°$and SDin in the postplacental hypoxia model was larger than those in the preplacental hypoxia and uteroplacental hypoxia model. Postplacental hypoxia would cause more varied displacement pattern than preplacental hypoxia and uteroplacental hypoxia.

According to the aforementioned results, postplacental hypoxia would have the small region displaced with various directions, and preplacental hypoxia and uteroplacental hypoxia would have the large region displaced with similar directions. In the intervillous space, the maternal blood in postplacental hypoxia might hardly circulate around the villous tree because of the small displacement regions with various directions while that in preplacental hypoxia and uteroplacental hypoxia might experience difficulties in circulation because of the large region displaced with similar directions. In the terminal villi, the fetal blood in postplacental hypoxia might have difficulty in circulation because the small amount of the capillaries would be received the displacement with various directions while that preplacental hypoxia and uteroplacental hypoxia might flow in the capillaries with difficulties because the large amount of the fetal blood would receive the displacement with similar directions.

The villous tree model enables us to depict the displacement pattern in the placenta, which is linked to the mechanical environment. It is possible to apply the mechanical environment to the computation about the model of the terminal villi, which is composed of the capillaries [29]. In the meantime, telocytes in the placenta have been found [30–33]. The distribution of the telocytes should be considered because the placenta is an innervated organ. Moreover, a novel medical imaging method available for the placenta [34] is also developed. If the villus tree model and the aforementioned findings and methods are combined together, dysfunctions in the placenta can be estimated more precisely.

5. Conclusion

In this chapter, how hypoxia influences the displacement caused by the contraction of the stem villi was estimated. Preplacental hypoxia and uteroplacental hypoxia would cause similar displacement directions in large regions while postplacental hypoxia would cause small displaced regions with various directions. Both of them might cause difficulties for the fetal and maternal circulations in the placenta.

Conflict of interest

None.

Author details

Yoko Kato

Address all correspondence to: ykato@mail.tohoku-gakuin.ac.jp

Faculty of Engineering, Tohoku Gakuin University, Tagajo, Miyagi, Japan

References

[1] Benirschke K, Burton GJ, Baergen RN. Pathology of the human placenta. 6th ed. Berlin Heidelberg: Springer-Verlag; 2012 . 941p. DOI: 10.1007/978-3-642-23941-0

[2] Illsley NP, Hall S, Stacey TE. The modulation of glucose transfer across the human placenta by intervillous flow rates: An in vitro perfusion study. Trophoblast Research. 1987;**2**:535-544

[3] Lofthouse EM, Perazzolo S, Brooks S, Crocker IP, Glazier JD, Johnstone ED, Panitchob N, Sibley CP, Widdows KL, Sengers BG, Lewis RM. Phenylalanine transfer across the isolated perfused human placenta: Experimental and modelling investigation. American Journal of Physiology. Regulatory, Integrative and Comparative Physiology. 2015; **310**(9):R828-R836. DOI: 10.1152/ajpregu.00405.2015

[4] Todros T, Sciarrone A, Piccoli E, Guiot C, Kaufmann P, Kingdom J. Umbilical Doppler waveforms and placental villous angiogenesis in pregnancies complicated by fetal growth restriction. Obstetrics and Gynecology. 1999;**93**(4):499-503. DOI: 10.1016/S0029-7844(98)00440-2

[5] Todros T, Piccoli E, Rolfo A, Cardropoli S, Guiot C, Gaglioti P, Oberto M, Vasario E, Canigga I. Review: Feto-placental vascularization: A multifaceted approach. Placenta.

2011;**32**(Supplement B, Trophoblast Research Vol. 25):S165-S169. DOI: 10.1016/j.placenta.2010.12.020

[6] Brunelli R, Masselli G, Parasassi T, De Spirito M, Papi M, Perrone G, Pittaluga E, Gualdi G, Pollettini E, Pittalis A, Anceschi MM. Intervillous circulation in intra-uterine growth restriction. Correlation to fetal well being. Placenta. 2010;**31**:1051-1056. DOI: 10.1016/j.placenta.2010.09.004

[7] Huen I, Morris DM, Wright C, Parker GJM, Sibley CP, Johnstone ED, Naish JH. R1 and R2* changes in the human placenta in response to maternal oxygen challenge. Magnetic Resonance in Medicine. 2013;**70**(5):1422-1433. DOI: 10.1002/mrm.24581

[8] Raine-Fening NJ, Campbell BK, Clewes JS, Kendall NR, Johnson IR. The reliability of virtual organ computer-aided analysis (VOCAL) for the semi quantification of ovarian, endometrical and subendometrial perfusion. Ultrasound in Obstetrics & Gynecology. 2003;**22**:633-639. DOI: 10.1002/uog.923

[9] Morel O, Grangé G, Fresson J, Schaaps JP, Foidart JM, Cabrol D, Tsatsaris V. Vascularization of the placenta and the subplacental myometrium: feasibility and reproducibility of a three-dimensional power Doppler ultrasound quantification technique. A pilot study. The Journal of Maternal-Fetal & Neonatal Medicine. 2011;**24**(2):284-290. DOI: 10.3109/14767058.2010.486845

[10] Kaufmann P, Sen DK, Schweikhart G. Classification of human placental villi: I. Histology. Cell and Tissue Research. 1979;**200**:409-423. DOI: 10.1007/BF00234852

[11] Leiser R, Luckhardt M, Kaufmann P, Winterhager E, Bruns U. The fetal vascularizsation of term human placental villi. I. Peripheral stem villi. Anatomy and Embryology (Berlin). 1985;**173**(1):71-80. DOI: 10.1007/BF00707305

[12] Kaufmann P, Bruns U, Leiser R, Luckhardt M, Winterhager E. The fetal vascularisation of term human placental villi. II. Intermediate and terminal villi. Anatomy and Embryology (Berlin). 1985;**173**(2):203-214. DOI: 10.1007/BF00316301

[13] Happe H. Beobachtungen an eihäuten junger menschlicher eier [Observation at embryonic membranes of early human embryos]. Anatomische Hefte. 1906;**32**(2):172-212

[14] Krantz KE, Parker JC. Contractile properties of the smooth muscle in the human placenta. Clinical Obstetrics and Gynecology. 1963;**6**:6-38

[15] Graf R, Langer JU, Schönfelder G, Öney T, Hartel-Schenk S, Reuter W, Schmidt HHHW. The extravascular contractile system in the human placenta: Morphological and immunocytochemical investigations. Anatomy and Embryology (Berlin). 1994;**190**:541-548. DOI: 10.1007/BF00190104

[16] Graf R, Schönfelder G, Mühlberger M, Gutsann M. The perivascular contractile sheath of human placental stem villi: Its isolation and characterization. Placenta. 1995;**16**:57-66. DOI: 10.1016/0143-4004(95)90081-0

[17] Graf R, Neudeck H, Gossrau R, Vetter K. Elastic fibres are an essential component of human placental stem villous stroma and an integrated part of the perivascular contractile sheath. Cell and Tissue Research. 1996;**283**:131-141. DOI: 10.1007/s004410050521

[18] Kohnen G, Kertschanska S, Demir R, Kaufmann P. Placental villous stroma as a model system for myofibroblast differentiation. Histochemistry and Cell Biology. 1996;**105**:415-429. DOI: 10.1007/BF01457655

[19] Graf R, Matetjevic D, Schuppan D, Neudeck H, Shakibaei M, Vetter K. Molecular anatomy of the perivascular sheath in human placental stem villi: The contractile apparatus and its association to the extracellular matrix. Cell and Tissue Research. 1997;**290**:601-607. DOI: 10.1007/s004410050965

[20] Demir R, Kosanke G, Kohnen G, Kertschanska S, Kaufmann P. Classification of human placental stem villi: Review of structural and functional aspects. Microscopy Research and Technique. 1997;**38**:28-41. DOI: 10.1002/(SICI)1097-0029(19970701/15)38:1/2<29::AID-JEMT5>3.0.CO;2-P

[21] Farley AE, Graham CH, Smith GN. Contractile properties of human placental anchoring villi. American Journal of Physiology. Regulatory, Integrative and Comparative Physiology. 2004;**287**:R680-R684. DOI: 10.1152/ajpregu.00222.2004

[22] Lecarpentier E, Claes V, Timbely O, Hébert JL, Arsalane A, Moumen A, Guerin C, Guizard M, Michel F, Lecarpentier Y. Role of both actin-myosin cross bridges and NO-cGMP pathway modulators in the contraction and relaxation of human placental stem villi. Placenta. 2013;**34**:1163-1169. DOI: 10.1016/j.placenta.2013.10.007

[23] Lecarpentier Y, Claes V, Lecarpentier E, Guerin C, Hébert JL, Arsalane A, Moumen A, Krokidis X, Michel F, Timbely O. Ultraslow myosin molecular motors of placental contractile stem villi in humans. PLoS One. 2014;**9**:e108814. DOI: 10.1371/journal.pone.0108814

[24] Kato Y, Oyen ML, Burton GJ. Villous tree model with active contractions for estimating blood flow conditions in the human placenta. The Open Biomedical Engineering Journal. 2017;**11**:36-48. DOI: 10.2174/1874120701711010036

[25] Kaufmann P, Luckhardt M, Shweikhart G, Cantle SJ. Cross-sectional features and three-dimensional structure of human placental villi. Placenta. 1987;**8**:235-247. DOI: 10.1016/0143-4004(87)90047-6

[26] Kingdom JCP, Kaufmann P. Oxygen and placental villous development: Origin of fetal hypoxia. Placenta. 1997;**18**:613-621. DOI: 10.1016/S0143-4004(97)90000-X

[27] Kato Y, Oyen ML, Burton GJ. Placental villous tree models for evaluating the mechanical environment in the human placenta. In: Proceedings of the 2014 IEEE International Conference on Imaging Systems and Techniques (IST); 14-17 October 2014; Santrini. IEEE; 2014. pp. 107-111. DOI: 10.1109/IST.2014.6958455

[28] Todros T, Marzioni D, Lorenzi T, Piccoli E, Capparuccia L, Perugini V, Cardaropoli S, Romagnoli R, Gesuita R, Rolfo A, Paulesu L, Castelluci M. Evidence for a role of TGF-β1 in the expression and regulation of α-SMA in fetal growth restricted placentae. Placenta. 2007;**28**:1123-1132. DOI: 10.1016/j.placenta.2007.06.003

[29] Pearce P, Brownbill P, Janáček J, Jirkovská M, Kubínová L, Chernyavsky L, Jensen OE. Image-based modeling of blood flow and oxygen transfer in feto-placental cappilaries. PLoS One. 2016;**11**(10):e165369. DOI: 10.1371/journal.pone.0165369

[30] Suciu L, Popescu LM, Gherghiceanu M. Human plcaenta: *de visu* demonstration of interstitial Cajal-like cells. Journal of Cellular and Molecular Medicine. 2007;**11**(3):590-597. DOI: 10.1111/j.1582-4934.2007.00058.x

[31] Popescu LM, Faussone-Pellegrini MSF. Telocytes—A case of serendipity: The winding way from interstitial cells of Cajal (ICC) *via* interstitial Cajal-like cells (ICLC) to telocytes. Journal of Cellular and Molecular Medicine. 2010;**14**(4):729-740. DOI: 10.1111/j.1582-4934.2010.01059.x

[32] Bosco C, Díaz. Presence of telocytes in a non-innervated organ: The placenta. In: Wang X, Cretoiu E, editors. Telocytes–Connecting Cells (Advances in Experimental Medicine and Biology). Singapore: Springer Science+Business Media Singapore; 2016. pp. 149-161. DOI: 10.1007/978-981-10-1061-3

[33] Nizyaeva NV, Sukhacheva TV, Serov RA, Kulikova GV, Nagovitsyna MN, Kan NE, Tyutyunnik VL, Pavlovich SV, Poltavtseva RA, Yarotskaya EL, Shchegolev AI, Sukhikh GT. Ultrastructural and immunohistochemical features of telocytes in placental villi in preeclampsia. Scientific Reports. 2018;**8**:3453. DOI: 10.1038/s41598-018-21492-w

[34] Hasegawa J, Suzuki N. SMI for imaging of placental infarction. Placenta. 2016;**47**:96-98. DOI: 10.1016/J.placenta.2016.08.092

Chapter 4

Cerebral Hemodynamics in Pediatric Hydrocephalus: Evaluation by Means of Transcranial Doppler Sonography

Branislav Kolarovszki

Additional information is available at the end of the chapter

http://dx.doi.org/10.5772/intechopen.79559

Abstract

Active, progressive hydrocephalus in children leads to increase of intracranial pressure, dilatation of cerebral ventricles, and decrease of intracranial compliance. These changes lead to disorder of regulation of cerebral circulation and development of cerebral hypoperfusion resulting in the secondary brain damage. Ependymal disruption, periventricular edema, and compression of the periventricular capillaries can be developed. Ischemia of the white matter can be developed due to hypoperfusion. But it is reversible if treated early and adequately. Transcranial Doppler sonography enables to determine hemodynamic parameters of cerebral circulation in various physiological and pathophysiological conditions. As transcranial Doppler sonography has been regarded to be noninvasive and appropriate for bedside treatment, it can also be applied in children at any age. The goal of this chapter is to assess changes of cerebral circulation in children with hydrocephalus and application of data from scientific studies of intracranial dynamics in children with hydrocephalus in clinical practice. The work is also focused on evaluation of impact of intracranial factors on Doppler parameters of cerebral circulation, especially in neonates with hydrocephalus. The ambition of this chapter is to improve indication and timing of drainage procedure in children with hydrocephalus by application of the results and clinical experience in daily clinical practice.

Keywords: cerebral hemodynamics, transcranial Doppler sonography, pediatric hydrocephalus

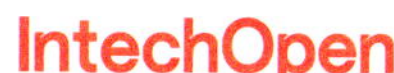

1. Introduction

Increased accumulation of cerebrospinal fluid in children with hydrocephalus leads to increased intracranial pressure, dilatation of the cerebral ventricles, decrease of intracranial compliance, and reduction of the brain tissue with negative impact on neurological condition of the child and his neurological development in the future. Alteration of cerebral circulation includes compression of the cerebral capillaries, stretching of the cerebral arteries, dysregulation of cerebral circulation, increase of cerebrovascular resistance, and decrease of cerebral blood flow. Progression of damage of the brain tissue results from decrease of blood flow in the brain and cerebral ischemia accompanied by changes in energetic metabolism. To measure the acute reversible cerebrovascular changes, and thus improve indication and timing of drainage procedure in noninvasive way, there is a need for examination technique, which could be used in daily clinical practice. This is the potential of transcranial Doppler sonography. It can analyze blood flow in the cerebral arteries and thus enables to perform noninvasive assessment of hemodynamic parameters of cerebral circulation.

Interpretation of changes in the Doppler curve of the cerebral arteries in pediatric hydrocephalus remains to be a discussed issue. Increase of cerebrovascular resistance of the cerebral arteries due to increased intracranial pressure is reflected in change of blood flow velocity and increased values of qualitative indices in the Doppler curve. Generally, there is good correlation between resistance index and pulsatility index of the cerebral arteries and intracranial pressure. Relationship between intracranial pressure, clinical manifestations of intracranial hypertension, dilatation of the cerebral ventricles, and Doppler parameters of the cerebral arteries is defined by biomechanical properties of the cranium and the brain in various age groups in children. It may be also influenced by many intra- and extracranial factors, which affect cerebral circulation [1]. In critically ill children, several factors are usually combined, which may, but do not have to, affect changes in the Doppler curve of the cerebral arteries. Therefore, cerebral blood flow in this type of patients has to be assessed carefully.

2. Doppler parameters of cerebral circulation in pediatric hydrocephalus

Bada et al. [2] were the first who described *the relationship between Doppler parameters of cerebral circulation and intracranial pressure* in preterm neonates with posthemorrhagic hydrocephalus. The results showed increased resistance index of the cerebral arteries due to increased intracranial pressure [2]. In the same year, Hill and Vople [3] presented results of their research on changes of RI-ACA in neonates with hydrocephalus. In nine out of ten cases, dilatation of the cerebral ventricles was accompanied by increase of intracranial pressure. In all cases, RI-ACA was increased. It was affected mainly by decrease of Ved. After drainage procedure, RI-ACA decreased due to increase of Ved. According to the authors, ventriculomegaly was considered more significant factor influencing hemodynamic parameters of ACA than increased intracranial pressure. Because in most of the cases, dilatation of the cerebral ventricles was accompanied by increased intracranial pressure, it is difficult to differentiate impact of dilatation of the cerebral ventricles from impact of increased intracranial pressure on cerebral circulation [3].

Fisher and Livingstone [4] observed change of parameters of blood flow in the Doppler curve in MCA, ACA, and ICA. The research revealed increase of PI, significant decrease of Ved, and slight decrease of Vsyst before drainage procedure. After drainage procedure, in which functional internal drainage system had been applied, return of hemodynamic parameters to normal range of values was confirmed. However, this change was not accompanied by return of size of the cerebral ventricles to standard values, excluding width of the third cerebral ventricle. Correlation between size of the cerebral ventricles and Vsyst was not proven. Relationship between Ved and size of the cerebral ventricle was intraindividual in its nature. The strongest correlation was measured between size of the cerebral ventricles and pulsatility index. Regarding morphological parameters, width of the third cerebral ventricle showed to be a precise indicator of changes of intracranial volume [4]. It was found out that ACA and MCA have the highest predisposition to early reaction to change of intracranial dynamics [4, 5]. During observation of RI-ACA, RI-MCA and RI-ICA in children with hydrocephalus before drainage procedure as well as in the early and later postsurgical period, the biggest changes of blood flow Doppler parameters were found in the anterior cerebral artery [6]. In children with hydrocephalus, Nishimaki et al. [7] measured RI-ACA and RI-BA. They found out that both indices were significantly increased before drainage procedure, but RI-ACA was more increased than RI-BA. However, indices of both cerebral arteries were significantly increased after drainage procedure, and decrease of RI-ACA was more significant than RI-BA. Significant change of RI-ACA comparing with change of RI-BA before and after drainage procedure is probably determined by anatomical location of the arteries. The anterior artery lies closely to the lateral cerebral ventricles and the third cerebral ventricle, and the basilar artery is located in the basilar cistern in front of the pons. In most of the cases of hydrocephalus, the lateral cerebral ventricles dilate more than the third and the fourth cerebral ventricles. Therefore, the authors of the study assume that dilatation of cerebral ventricles has greater effect on the anterior cerebral ventricle than on the basilar artery [7].

Although the basilar artery does not belong to the arteries with the highest predisposition to early reaction to volume-pressure changes in the intracranial space, assessment of increased RI-BA value and size of the cerebral ventricles, which had been performed in dogs with hydrocephalus, helped to distinguish cases, in which drainage procedure is necessary—with sensitivity of 77% and specificity of 94%. The value of neurological manifestations of symptomatic hydrocephalus correlated with RI-BA value and size of the cerebral ventricles. During measurement of individual dynamics, changes in clinical symptomatology had been accompanied by changes of RI-BA and size of the cerebral ventricles [8].

When observing changes of pulsatility index and cerebral ventricles resistance in children with hydrocephalus before and after drainage procedure, various studies revealed significant increase of PI and RI values of the cerebral ventricles before drainage procedure and significant decrease of PI and RI in functional drainage internal system after surgery. Change of qualitative indices of the Doppler curve was affected by change of Ved. The results of studies showed that increased cerebrovascular resistance before drainage procedure was determined by increased intracranial pressure, which is reversible after drainage procedure. Positive impact of drainage procedure on Doppler parameters of the cerebral arteries is based on postsurgical change of cerebrovascular resistance and regulation of cerebral circulation due to decrease of intracranial pressure [6, 9–12]. Significant relationship between resistance index and pulsatility index of MCA was observed in infants with congenital hydrocephalus before the operation [13].

The assessment of Doppler parameters of cerebral circulation and heart rate variability in preterm neonates with posthemorrhagic hydrocephalus showed that hemodynamic parameters as well as chronotropic regulation of cardiac function changed after drainage procedure [14].

On the contrary, van Bel et al. [15], who investigated ten preterm neonates with posthemorrhagic hydrocephalus before drainage procedure, proved significant increase of PI-ACA resulting from significant increase of Vsyst. After successful performance of drainage procedure, PI-ACA and Vsyst significantly decreased. The values of PI-ACA after drainage of cerebrospinal fluid were within standard range. When van Bel et al. [15] compared values of Ved and Vmean before and after drainage procedure, they did not found any significant changes. It may be concluded that increase of PI-ACA before drainage procedure was determined only by increase of Vsyst [15]. The same results were confirmed by Alvisi et al. [18]. Many researchers claim that increase of Vsyst before drainage procedure is caused by movement and compression of the anterior cerebral arteries through enlarged cerebral ventricles and flow of cerebrospinal fluid into the white matter, which results in decrease of transmural pressure gradient [16–18].

In neonates, infants, and older children, Goh et al. [19, 20] studied relationship between intracranial pressure and resistance index of ACA and MCA. They found good intraindividual correlation between ICP and RI-ACA and RI-MCA in neonates and general good correlation between ICP and RI-ACA and RI-MCA in infants and older children. Difference between the age groups is probably caused by individual pressure-volume compensation of the intracranial pressure in neonates with hydrocephalus in various stages of hydrocephalus and various degree of compliance of the calva and cranial sutures. Intracranial dynamics is more uniform in infants and older children. This corresponds with general good correlation between intracranial pressure and resistance index of the cerebral arteries. Significant decrease of RI-ACA and RI-MCA, determined by increase of Ved, was observed after drainage procedure in all age categories. Only in neonates, increase of Ved was accompanied by moderate increase of Vsyst and Vmean [19, 20].

During continuous observation of blood flow in MCA by transcranial Doppler sonography, positive impact of drainage of cerebrospinal fluid on Doppler parameters of MCA had been observed in children with hydrocephalus during the insertion of ventriculoperitoneal shunt. Insertion of ventricular catheter into the lateral cerebral ventricle with cerebrospinal fluid derivation led to obvious and immediate 30% increase of blood flow in MCA. When drainage procedure had been performed, values of PI-MCA, which were increased before the surgery, returned to standard range. The results of the study confirmed positive impact of cerebrospinal fluid derivation on hemodynamic parameters of cerebral circulation in children with hydrocephalus [21].

Results of various studies emphasize the importance of data from assessment of changes of Doppler parameters of cerebral circulation to the monitoring of *dilatation of cerebral ventricles*. Experiment on newborn rats with progressive communicating hydrocephalus showed that onset of ventricular dilatation was not accompanied by alteration of parameters in the Doppler curve of the cerebral arteries. Pulsatility index of the cerebral arteries had been increased during development of hydrocephalus and followed by progression of ventricular dilatation. This means that dilatation of cerebral ventricles did not change pulsatility index of the cerebral arteries. Instead, the change occurred due to progression of hydrocephalus and increase of intracranial pressure. It can be concluded that in this developmental stage of hydrocephalus, cerebral circulation was more influenced by increased intracranial pressure than by ventricular dilatation [22]. In chronic stage, changes of cerebral hemodynamics and advanced ventricular dilatation were accompanied by other structural pathological changes [23].

Relation between *dynamics of ventricular dilatation* (progressive, stable, or regressive) and basal and compressive values of RI-ACA was not found in neonates with hydrocephalus before the drainage procedure. It means that dynamics of ventricular dilatation is not the only parameter influencing Doppler parameters of the cerebral arteries. In all cases of neonates with hydrocephalus, intracranial pressure was increased during drainage procedure, and clinical manifestations of intracranial hypertension had diminished after the surgery. Therefore, the authors of the study assume that Doppler parameters of the cerebral arteries are influenced by combination of increased intracranial pressure and ventricular dilatation. Additionally, the results of the study confirmed that not only progressive but also stable ventricular dilatation with increased intracranial pressure has negative effect on cerebral circulation [12]. On the contrary, in neonates with stable ventricular dilatation, in which drainage procedure was not necessary, basal Doppler parameters of blood flow in ACA reached normal values. Similarly, Quinn and Pople [24] confirmed increase of PI-MCA in children with hydrocephalus who experienced dysfunction of drainage system. CT examination, however, revealed change of size of the lateral ventricles only in 10 out of 32 patients. Comparing with stable ventricular dilatation, results showed increased value of PI-MCA and the presence of clinical manifestations of dysfunction of drainage system, in which surgical procedure is necessary. When the procedure had been performed, PI-MCA significantly decreased [24]. However, if intracranial pressure was not increased in stable ventricular dilatation, resistance index of the cerebral ventricles did not change either [25].

Not only increase of intracranial pressure and development of ventricular dilatation but also changes of the cerebral arteries, such as distortion, compression, and stretching may occur in children with hydrocephalus [26].

The results of the study Kolarovszki et al. [12] on children with hydrocephalus confirmed that *asymmetric ventricular dilatation* had significantly influenced values of basal RI-ACA before drainage procedure and compressive RI-ACA after it. Statistical analysis showed that values of basal RI-ACA after drainage procedure and compressive RI-ACA before drainage procedure were not influenced by asymmetric ventricular dilatation. Asymmetric ventricular dilatation before drainage procedure may lead to stretching of the anterior cerebral arteries. When accompanied by increased intracranial pressure, it results in increase of cerebrovascular resistance and RI-ACA value. The presumption that asymmetry of the cerebral ventricle has significant impact on presurgical values of compressive RI-ACA was not confirmed. The authors believe that it was caused by distribution of range of compressive RI-ACA before drainage procedure. In 36 neonates out of 40 (90%), compressive RI-ACA before drainage procedure reached maximal value of 1.0 regardless asymmetric ventricular dilatation. In normal values of intracranial pressure measured after drainage procedure, the values of basal RI-ACA were not influenced by asymmetric ventricular dilatation. In cases with standard values of intracranial pressure in asymmetric ventricular dilatation, dislocation of the anterior cerebral ventricles may occur without significant stretching and change of cerebrovascular resistance. Compression of the anterior fontanelle in asymmetric ventricular dilatation, which is related to intracranial normotension, may worsen dislocation of the anterior cerebral ventricles if it is accompanied by increase of cerebrovascular resistance resulting in compressive RI-ACA. Based on the study and clinical experience, the authors emphasize the fact that interpretation of Doppler parameters of the cerebral arteries in pediatric hydrocephalus with asymmetry of cerebral ventricles has to be done carefully [12].

In neonates with hydrocephalus, besides hydrocephalus itself, the following pathological changes of the periventricular cerebral tissue may also have negative impact on cerebral circulation: periventricular leukomalacia and peri- and intraventricular hemorrhage.

Impact of these changes on cerebral circulation and Doppler parameters of the cerebral arteries should be taken into consideration when assessing hemodynamic parameters of cerebral circulation in neonates with hydrocephalus in relation to observation of intracranial dynamics and indication of drainage procedure.

In neonates with hydrocephalus, besides hydrocephalus itself, the following pathological changes of the periventricular cerebral tissue may also have negative impact on cerebral circulation: periventricular leukomalacia and peri- and intraventricular hemorrhage. Impact of these changes on cerebral circulation and Doppler parameters of the cerebral arteries should be taken into consideration when assessing hemodynamic parameters of cerebral circulation in neonates with hydrocephalus in relation to observation of intracranial dynamics and indication of drainage procedure.

The most common cause of *periventricular leukomalacia* is perinatal infection (e.g., chorioamnionitis) and hypoxic-ischemic damage of the brain tissue. Considering various degrees of maturity of the brain tissue, consequences of hypoxic-ischemic brain injury differ in preterm neonates and term neonates [27].

In preterm neonates, the periventricular white matter is at higher risk of hypoxia, which leads to focal or diffuse type of periventricular leukomalacia, while in term neonates, it is the white matter near the cerebral cortex, in which cortical or subcortical lesions of white matter can be detected [28].

The cystic leukomalacia lesions do not occur from the moment of primary insult of the brain tissue, but they develop continuously. At first, hyperechogenicity of the periventricular brain tissue is confirmed by a sonography. Then cystic lesions are formed during 10–14 days [29]. Pathological changes of structure of the periventricular brain tissue are accompanied by hemodynamic changes. Dysfunction of cerebral autoregulation was confirmed in preterm neonates with periventricular leukomalacia [30]. Many researchers also confirmed alteration of cerebral circulation in neonates with periventricular leukomalacia. By means of transcranial Doppler ultrasonography, Fukuda et al. observed long-term decrease of blood flow velocity within all major cerebral arteries [31]. In another research on periventricular leukomalacia in neonates with low birth weight, Fukuda et al. confirmed that blood flow in ICA and VA had decreased a few days after birth and then between day 21 and 42 [32]. Research by Ilves et al. [33] revealed that mean velocity of blood flow in ACA, MCA, ICA, and BA had increased in 83 asphyctic term

http://dx.doi.org/10.5772/intechopen.79559

neonates due to severe hypoxic-ischemic encephalopathy during first days after asphyxia. However, increased mean velocity of blood flow in the cerebral arteries was only short term. During period of 21–59 days, it dropped below standard values of healthy term neonates [33]. Changes of Doppler parameters of MCA in neonates with hypoxic-ischemic encephalopathy were also proven by Liu et al. [34]. In children with severe encephalopathy, the values of RI-MCA were < 0.50 or RI-MCA > 0.90 as a result of change of blood flow velocity in MCA.

To classify *intracranial hemorrhage in neonates*, the grading scale of Papile, which was created in 1978, is still being used [35]. In the past, it was assumed that the grade IV denotes spread of subependymal bleeding into the surrounding brain tissue. Nowadays, decrease of venous drainage and development of venous hemorrhagic infarction are regarded to be the main triggers of intracranial hemorrhage in neonates [27, 36]. Subsequently, porencephalic cysts may develop in the site of periventricular venous infarction. In general, higher grades of intracranial hemorrhage lead to increased risk of severe neurological disorders in children. If degrees III and IV of intracranial hemorrhage occur in active hydrocephalus, the brain tissue and cerebral circulation of a neonate are negatively affected by bleeding itself as well as changes related to intracranial pressure and progressive dilatation of cerebral ventricles. Moreover, there are many extracranial factors, which impact negatively on cerebral circulation, especially in preterm neonates [37–39].

Peri- and intracranial hemorrhage in neonates leads to dysfunction of regulation of cerebral circulation including autoregulation. Increased values of resistance index of the cerebral arteries, which were found out in the site of bleeding, are a sign of increased cerebrovascular resistance and presence of vasoconstriction near hemorrhagic lesions [40, 41]. Various research studies on neonates with posthemorrhagic hydrocephalus showed positive effect of drainage procedures, decrease of intracranial pressure, and the improvement of cerebral circulation.

The issue of frequency and appropriate time management of cerebrospinal fluid derivation during intermittent drainage in neonates with posthemorrhagic hydrocephalus remains open to debate. Large multicentric studies confirmed very low effect of frequent and early performed drainage, based on the assessment of size of the cerebral ventricles, in comparison with a conservative approach [42]. Since one of the prospective goals of intermittent drainage of cerebrospinal fluid is to prevent dysfunction of cerebral circulation due to increased intracranial pressure, changes of Doppler parameters of cerebral circulation in neonates with posthemorrhagic hydrocephalus have become a center of attention.

Nishimaki et al. [43] found out values of RI-ACA in children with posthemorrhagic hydrocephalus were significantly increased before lumbar puncture or puncture of subcutaneous reservoir. But after aspiration of 5–10 ml/kg, they significantly decreased [43]. Similarly, Kempley and Gamsu [44] confirmed decrease of intracranial pressure accompanied by significant increase of Vmean and decrease of PI-ACA, when cerebrospinal fluid derivation had been performed in newborn with posthemorrhagic hydrocephalus. Quinn et al. [45] compared impact of increased intracranial pressure and cerebrospinal fluid derivation on blood flow in ACA and ICV in neonates with posthemorrhagic hydrocephalus. RI-ACA was significantly increased before drainage procedure. But afterward, it decreased significantly. Changes of blood flow velocity in ACA were not accompanied by change of blood flow velocity in ICV [45].

Maertzdorf et al. [46] observed hemodynamic parameters of ACA and MCA in the Doppler curve of preterm neonates with intraventricular hemorrhage and posthemorrhagic hydrocephalus during early gestation weeks. Aspirations of cerebrospinal fluid from subcutaneous reservoir of the ventricular catheter (type Ommaya) had been performed repetitively. When ICP before drainage procedure was ≥6 cm H_2O, then Ved and Vmean had increased significantly after performing aspiration. When ICP was <6 cm H_2O, RI-ACA and RI-MCA had decreased. Value of Vsyst was significantly changing after cerebrospinal aspiration. The results confirmed good intraindividual correlation between RI-ACA, RI-MCA, and ICP in neonates with posthemorrhagic hydrocephalus [46]. The use of near-infrared spectroscopy revealed that cerebrospinal fluid derivation from subcutaneous reservoir lead not only to change of Doppler parameters of cerebral circulation, especially significant decrease of pulsatility index, but also to improvement of intravascular oxygenation of cerebral circulation [47, 48].

During assessment of effect of periventricular posthemorrhagic lesions on Doppler parameters of blood flow in ACA of neonates with hydrocephalus, significant correlation had been found between periventricular posthemorrhagic lesions and basal RI-ACA and compressive RI-ACA after drainage procedure. Before drainage procedure, Doppler parameters in ACA were influenced by increased intracranial pressure and posthemorrhagic lesions [12].

Based on the research, it can be concluded that cerebrospinal fluid derivation in neonates with posthemorrhagic hydrocephalus leads to improvement of cerebral blood flow. While indicating and planning derivation of cerebrospinal fluid, changes of Doppler parameters of cerebral circulation should be taken into account [1] (**Figure 1**).

Changes of Doppler parameters of the cerebral arteries were found also in cases with *dysfunction of drainage system* after surgical revision in children with hydrocephalus.

Pople [49] focused on identification of referential values of PI-MCA in children with hydrocephalus with functional internal drainage system (**Table 1**). The sample included 248 asymptomatic children with hydrocephalus with functional shunt system. They were 1 week to 16 years old. It is known that blood flow velocity in the cerebral arteries increases during aging. Changes of blood flow velocity in the cerebral arteries are more variable in children, especially in younger age groups, than in adults. The highest blood flow velocity was measured between 3 and 4 years of age. Since then it had been gradually decreasing to the level of values in adults. Pulsatility index had been significantly decreasing during the first 6 months of age. The lowest value was measured between 2 and 6 years of age. Since then it had been gradually increasing up to the value of 0.9 in the age of 16. In addition to identification of referential values of PI-MCA in children with hydrocephalus with functional internal drainage system, Pople emphasized significant interindividual differences of Doppler parameters and importance of following the intraindividual trend [49]. In 63 children with hydrocephalus with dysfunction of drainage system, values of PI-MCA were compared with referential values. It was found out that increase of PI-MCA determines shunt malfunction with sensitivity of 56% and specificity of 97%. The values of PI-MCA correlated with intracranial pressure of children with shunt obstruction [50]. Increased resistance index of the cerebral arteries was also confirmed in children with dysfunction of drainage systems [12, 51] (**Figure 2**).

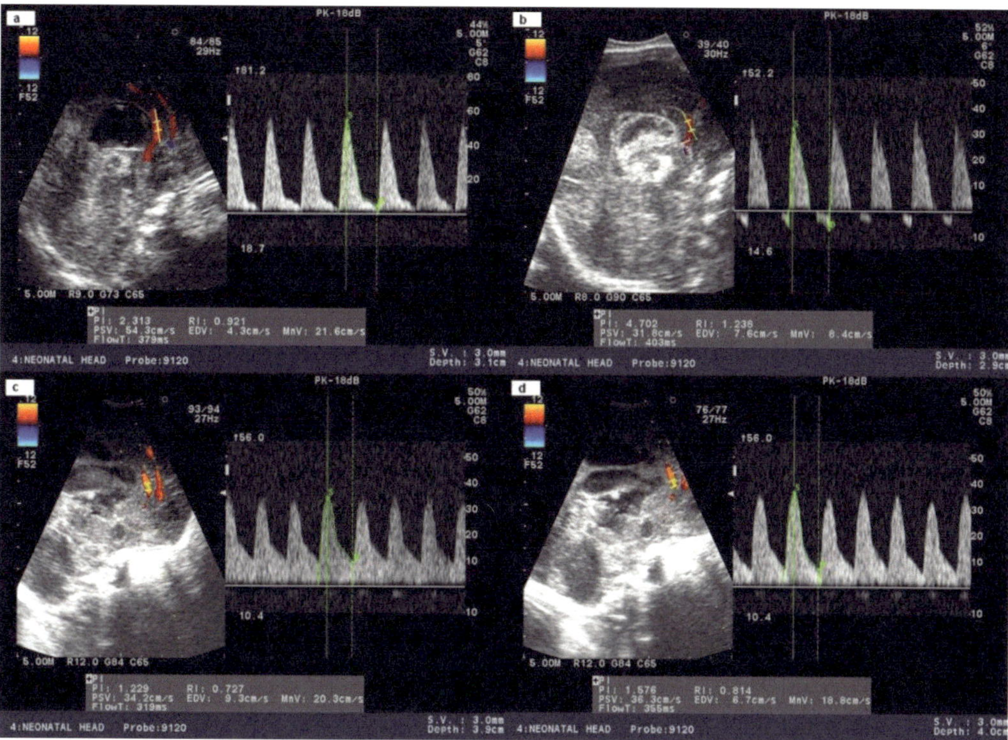

Figure 1. Doppler parameters of blood flow in the arteria cerebri anterior in the preterm neonate with posthemorrhagic hydrocephalus before and after drainage procedure. (a) Basal parameters before drainage procedure (increased RI, decreased Ved), (b) positive compressive test of the anterior fontanelle before drainage procedure (reverse blood flow during diastole), (c) basal parameters after drainage procedure (normal values of RI and Ved), and (d) negative compressive test of the anterior fontanelle after drainage procedure. Abbreviations used in the picture: RI, resistance index; Ved, end-diastolic velocity of blood flow; Vsyst, maximal systolic velocity of blood flow; PI, pulsatility index; Vmean, mean velocity of blood flow (figure—author).

Age	Vsyst (cm/s) (mean)	Ved (cm/s) (mean)	Vmean (cm/s) (mean)	Pulsatility index (mean)	Number (n = 248)
0–3 months	19–107 (63)	3–43 (23)	8–64 (36)	0.83–1.62 (1.23)	16
4–6 months	40–124 (82)	18–50 (34)	25–73 (49)	0.77–1.26 (1.01)	11
7–12 months	25–165 (95)	7–71 (39)	14–110 (62)	0.67–1.20 (0.94)	15
1–2 years	58–166 (112)	28–84 (56)	47–113 (75)	0.66–1.02 (0.82)	26
2–6 years	62–170 (116)	28–92 (60)	42–122 (82)	0.48–0.99 (0.74)	77
6–10 years	47–155 (101)	23–79 (51)	37–107 (67)	0.55–1.00 (0.77)	61
10–16 years	37–153 (95)	20–72 (56)	24–96 (60)	0.59–1.22 (0.89)	42

Table 1. Referential values of PI-MCA in children with hydrocephalus with functional internal drainage system [49].

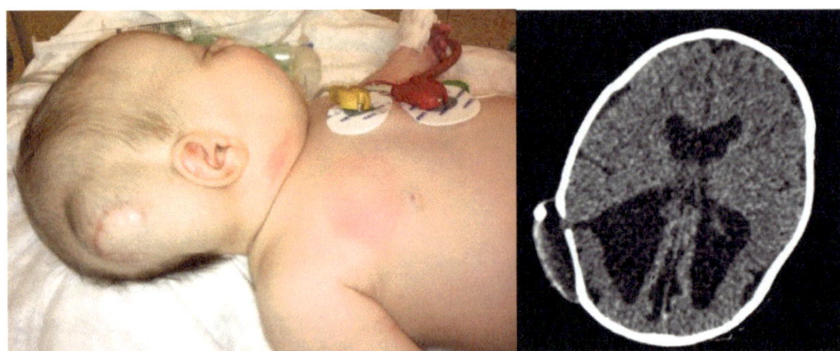

Figure 2. Dysfunction of ventriculoperitoneal shunt in the child with hydrocephalus. Manifestation of fistula and subcutaneous cerebrospinal fluid accumulation. CT image shows the dislocation of ventricular catheter from the intracranial space, fistula, and subcutaneous cerebrospinal fluid accumulation (figure—author).

Assessment of cerebral circulation by transcranial Doppler sonography can be used not only to observed functions of shunts but also ventriculostomy of the third cerebral ventricle. Vajda et al. [52] found out that PI-MCA significantly decreased in children with obstructive hydrocephalus after successful ETV. The difference was not statistically significant when they compared PI-MCA measured immediately after ETV with value measured in the fifth day after surgery. Effect of ventriculostomy was confirmed by assessment of cerebrospinal fluid flow using cine-phase MRI examination. Clinical symptomatology improved immediately after the procedure in 17 out of 22 patients. No correlation between PI-MCA and age or gender of children in the sample of patients was found. The results showed importance of Doppler sonography for observation of ETV functioning in the early postsurgical period [52].

In addition to increased resistance index of the cerebral arteries, vascular reactivity malfunction to p_aCO_2 change was detected in children with active hydrocephalus before drainage system insertion and in dysfunction of drainage system. When drainage system was inserted and dysfunctional shunt revised, resistance index decreased significantly. Then cerebrovascular reactivity to p_aCO_2 change had been improved and that also led to functional cerebral circulation and regulation change [53].

Taylor et al. [54] used *compressive test on the anterior fontanelle* during transcranial Doppler sonography examination in children with abnormal intracranial compliance. They studied basal values of RI-ACA and change of RI-ACA during the compressive test (**Figure 3**). The change was expressed as percentage difference in contrast to basal value. The basal values of RI-ACA of preterm neonates and neonates with abnormal intracranial compliance were significantly increased when compared to basal values of healthy term neonates. Only slight change of RI-MCA was observed in healthy preterm neonates and healthy term neonates during compression on the anterior fontanelle. However, RI-MCA was significantly increased in neonates with abnormal intracranial compliance. Basal values of RI-MCA were increased in neonates with increased intracranial pressure. Hemodynamic reaction of the cerebral vessels to compression of the anterior fontanelle had improved after drainage of cerebrospinal fluid. Compression test on the anterior fontanelle during transcranial Doppler sonography examination can help to detect alteration of intracranial compliance before increase of intracranial pressure. This is manifested

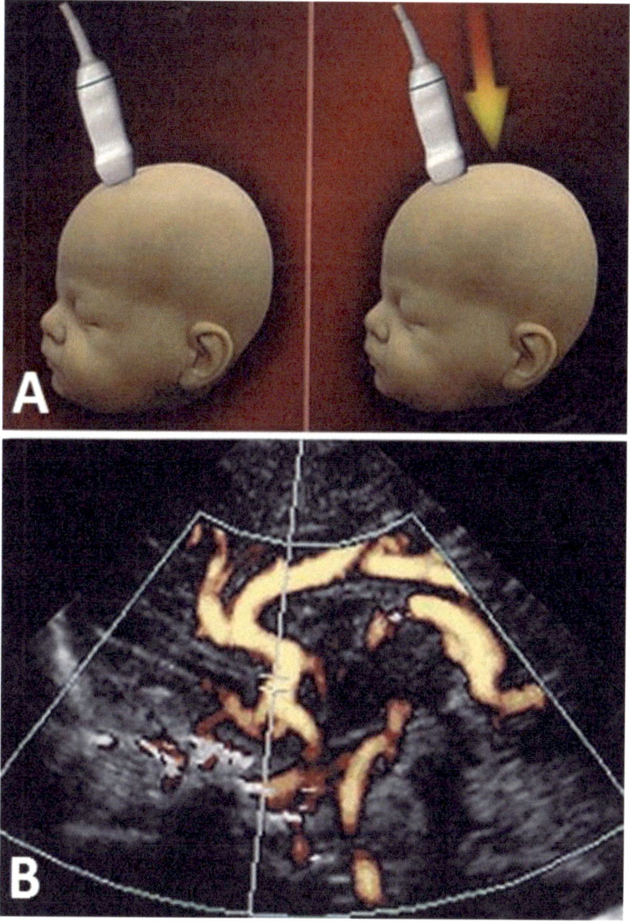

Figure 3. The compression test on the anterior fontanelle. (A) Compression by the sonographic probe and (B) the Doppler curve of the anterior cerebral artery [53].

by increased basal values of resistance index. The study showed possibility of indirect noninvasive measurement of intracranial compliance and intracranial pressure by transcranial Doppler sonography [54]. In another study, Taylor et al. [36] assessed hemodynamic reaction of the anterior cerebral artery during compressive test on the anterior fontanelle in neonates with hydrocephalus. The research was performed by means of compressive test. It revealed significant increase of RI-ACA in neonates who were indicated for drainage procedure and in which increased intracranial pressure was confirmed by direct measurement [36].

Westra et al. [55] also dealt with the use of compressive test on the anterior fontanelle in children with hydrocephalus. They confirmed significantly increased basal and also compressive values of RI-ACA in children hydrocephalus with increased intracranial pressure. Significant decrease of basal and compressive values of RI-ACA was found out when drainage procedure had been performed. Based on the results, they defined the boundary value of 0.70 for basal RI-ACA and 0.90 for compressive RI-ACA [55].

Gera et al. [56] focused on assessment of Doppler parameters of the anterior cerebral artery in relation to drainage procedure indication and change of measured Doppler parameters after drainage procedure. In children indicated for drainage procedure, they found out significantly increased value of basal RI-ACA and RI-ACA during compressive test. But after drainage procedure, the value of basal RI-ACA and compressive RI-ACA significantly decreased [56].

Change of Doppler parameters indicates increase of intracranial compliance after drainage procedure. However, no correlation between ICP and RI-ACA (both basal and compressive) was found. The researchers believe that it is caused by complexity of the relationship between ICP and RI and potential nonlinearity of the relationship. During observation of RI-ACA in children with hydrocephalus in relation to indication of drainage procedure, the following values of basal RI-ACA were found out: sensitivity of 72.5%, specificity of 80%, and diagnostic accuracy of 75%. Assessment of RI-ACA by compressive test on the anterior fontanelle showed sensitivity of 75%, specificity of 100%, and diagnostic accuracy of 83.3%. False negativity in assessment of basal and compressive RI-ACA was the same (25%). **Table 2** presents comparison of the role of assessment of hemodynamic parameters of the cerebral arteries by Doppler sonography during compressive test in children with hydrocephalus and indication of drainage system.

The compressive test on the anterior fontanelle increases sensitivity and specificity of resistance index and pulsatility index in regard to indirect measurement of increased intracranial pressure and decreased intracranial compliance in children with hydrocephalus. On the other hand, results of the compressive test require more careful assessment of effect of intra- and extracranial factors on cerebral circulation because their influence on compressive values is more significant than effect on basal values. Pressure applied to the anterior fontanelle during compressive test is defined within the range 0–200 g/cm^2. The pressure can gradually increase when using an ophtalmodynamometer [54]. When using a sonographic probe, shape (linear or convex) and size of a probe and pressure, which will be created by a doctor, need to be taken into consideration. Therefore, if a child was indicated for sonographic examination, it should be performed by the same doctor and the same probe. Regarding indirect measurement of intracranial hypertension and intracranial compliance, false positivity of compressive test can be found in preterm neonates who require intensive care (instability of extracranial factors), in severe stages of intra- and periventricular hemorrhage and ventricular dilatation. False negativity of compressive test can be caused by liquorea, subcutaneous cerebrospinal fluid fistula, or small size of the anterior fontanelle [12].

Although transcranial Doppler sonography has been used more than 30 years to assess Doppler parameters of cerebral circulation, interpretation of parameters in the Doppler curve of the

	Taylor [57] (%)	Westra et al. [55] (%)	Gera et al. [56] (%)
Sensitivity	45	81	75
Specificity	95	100	100

Table 2. The role of assessment of hemodynamic parameters of the cerebral arteries by Doppler sonography during compressive test in children with hydrocephalus and indication of drainage system.

cerebral arteries, intracranial pressure, intracranial compliance, and cerebral hemodynamics in children with hydrocephalus remains to be an open topic. On the one side, results of various studies showed possibility of indirect noninvasive assessment of intracranial pressure and compliance by means of transcranial Doppler sonography. On the other hand, results showed limitations and difficulties when assessing Doppler parameters of cerebral circulation in children with hydrocephalus. When assessing relation between intracranial pressure, resistance index, and pulsatility index of the cerebral vessels, wide range of factors, which can change shape and properties of the Doppler curve, need to be taken into consideration. Behrens et al. [58] used a mathematical model of cerebrospinal fluid circulation, which confirmed that relation between ICP and PI-MCA is significantly influenced by vascular compliance, autoregulation, and arterial pressure. They believe that individual variability of these physiological parameters is responsible for inaccurate reference of ICP value [58]. Similarly, Hanlo et al. [59] confirmed decreased resistance index and pulsatility index of the cerebral vessels measured in children with progressive hydrocephalus after drainage procedure. However, during longitudinal simultaneous ICP/transcranial Doppler sonography monitoring, correlation between ICP, RI, and PI was very weak. Based on the results, which showed wide range of referential Doppler parameters of cerebral circulation and impact of extracranial factors, authors of this study believe that pulsatility index and resistance index of the cerebral vessels do not help in assessment of intracranial dynamics in patients with increased intracranial pressure [59].

This inconsistency of results on assessment of relationship between RI and PI of the cerebral vessels, and intracranial pressure has led to research of more accurate noninvasive parameters of intracranial pressure. Hanlo et al. [59] presented new Doppler index known as trans-systolic time. The results confirmed that trans-systolic time of the cerebral arteries in the Doppler curve is less influenced by other factors (e.g., heart rate) and is more accurate for comparison of ICP, RI, and PI changes [60]. Also, Leliefeld et al. [61] confirmed significant correlation between trans-systolic time and ICP. Despite these positive results, assessments of trans-systolic time of the cerebral arteries are not used for noninvasive measurement of intracranial pressure. It might be caused by a lack of referential range in children population and lack of experience with use in clinical practice [61]. In another study, Leliefeld et al. [62] dealt with possibility to use MRI examination of cerebral circulation for indirect measurement of intracranial pressure. They found out that standard values of blood flow velocity in the brain and low values in ADC map were referred to compensated hydrocephalus without a need of drainage procedure. They claim that noninvasive changes of cerebral circulation by MRI examination enable to distinguish the cases of compensated children with hydrocephalus with standard intracranial pressure without a need of drainage procedure from the cases of gradually progressive hydrocephalus with a need of drainage surgery [62].

Galarza and Lazareff [63] focused on clinical validity of transcranial Doppler sonography in children with various types of hydrocephalus. The study showed that values of PI-MCA and RI-MCA were significantly higher in progressive hydrocephalus with a need of drainage procedure. On the other hand, RI-MCA and PI-MCA were not increased, and blood flow velocity in MCA was not decreased in the cases with compensated hydrocephalus (also known as arrested hydrocephalus) and ventriculomegaly (or essential ventriculomegaly). The results showed importance of transcranial Doppler sonography for indication of drainage procedure in children with hydrocephalus. However, the authors emphasize the importance of individual and careful assessment of Doppler parameters of cerebral circulation regarding children hydrocephalus in clinical practice [63].

Rodríguez-Nuñez et al. [64] confirmed the role of clinical manifestations of intracranial hypertension, radiological morphometric parameters of the brain (Evans' index), biochemical parameters of cerebrospinal fluid (level of hypoxanthine, xanthine, and urea acid), and Doppler parameters of the cerebral circulation during assessment of children hydrocephalus and indication of drainage procedure [64].

Based on the results of the works of several authors, it seems that *optic nerve sheath diameter (ONSD) ultrasonography* could be a good noninvasive method for the indirect detection of raised intracranial pressure [65–68].

The study of Ragauskas et al. [69] compared the diagnostic reliability of optic nerve sheath diameter ultrasonography with a transcranial Doppler sonography and the absolute values of intracranial pressure in neurological patients. The authors of this study found that the noninvasive ICP measurement method based on two-depth transcranial Doppler technology has a better diagnostic reliability on neurological patients than the ONSD method when expressed by the sensitivity and specificity for detecting elevated ICP >14.7 mmHg [69]. Tarzamni et al. [70] analyzed the diagnostic accuracy of ultrasonographic ONSD measurement and color Doppler indices of the ophthalmic arteries in detecting elevated intracranial pressure. While the ultrasonographic mean binocular ONSD was completely accurate in detecting elevated ICP, color Doppler indices of the ophthalmic arteries were of limited value [70].

Based on the recent literature, it seems to be a good idea to use sonographic methods, optic nerve sheath diameter ultrasonography and transcranial Doppler sonography for the noninvasive detection of intracranial hypertension. Further research for the application in clinical practice in pediatric hydrocephalus is needed.

3. Conclusion

Based on the clinical experience and scientific research on pediatric hydrocephalus, we can summarize the role of transcranial Doppler sonography in assessment of cerebral circulation and intracranial dynamics of pediatric hydrocephalus as follows:

1. Assessment of Doppler parameters of cerebral circulation before drainage procedure in children with hydrocephalus revealed alteration of cerebral circulation which is potentially reversible. Doppler sonography showed the improvement of cerebral circulation after the drainage procedure in pediatric hydrocephalus.
2. Results of compressive test on the anterior fontanelle increase validity of assessment of cerebral circulation by transcranial Doppler sonography and enable indirect assessment of decrease of intracranial compliance. Increase of basal Doppler parameters shows increase of intracranial pressure.

3. While interpreting Doppler parameters of cerebral circulation measured in a child with hydrocephalus, it is important to assess impact of both intra- and extracranial factors on cerebral circulation. Then it is possible to say to which extent Doppler parameters show the real value of intracranial pressure and intracranial compliance. The results showed that asymmetric dilatation of the lateral cerebral ventricles and posthemorrhagic periventricular lesions influence Doppler parameters of cerebral arteries both in intracranial hypertension and normotension.

4. The results show that the Doppler parameters of cerebral arteries in active hydrocephalus are not increased due to dilatation of cerebral ventricles but increased intracranial pressure.

5. Assessment of Doppler parameters of blood flow in cerebral arteries in children with hydrocephalus with functional drainage system or ETV revealed standard range of values. On the other hand, the values of Doppler parameters increased in the shunt-dependent children with dysfunctional drainage system or ETV, even though the cerebral ventricles enlarged slightly or maintained the same size. After successful revision surgery, the value of Doppler parameters dropped down to standard range.

6. Assessment of cerebral circulation by transcranial Doppler sonography in children with hydrocephalus can be easily performed by an accessible, indirect, noninvasive, bedside, and repetitive measurement of intracranial pressure and intracranial compliance. Regarding complexity of intracranial dynamics, relationship between intracranial pressure and Doppler parameters of the cerebral arteries, individual assessment of measured Doppler parameters, as well as assessment of effect of extra- and intracranial factors to cerebral circulation should be performed in each case of pediatric hydrocephalus. If the results are not clear, examination should be repeated, and intraindividual tendency should be observed in the child. It is important to design and follow detailed methodology of sonographic examination and include it into the report of assessment of intracranial dynamics in the child with hydrocephalus.

7. Clinical applications of transcranial Doppler sonography in pediatric hydrocephalus are as follows:

   - Indication and timing of drainage procedure;
   - Monitoring of effectivity of drainage procedure—internal drainage systems (shunts), ETV, external ventricular drainage, and cerebrospinal fluid derivation from subcutaneous reservoir (determination of frequency and amount of aspired cerebrospinal fluid);
   - Monitoring of function and detection of malfunction of external and internal drainage systems and ETV;
   - Assessment of the dependence of the child on drainage system (shunt-dependence)—important for indication of external ventricular drainage or subcutaneous reservoir conversion on internal drainage system (shunt) or ETV, need for a revision of dysfunctional drainage system.

To sum up, it can be said that including assessment of cerebral circulation by transcranial Doppler sonography into management of child with hydrocephalus provides additional information to clinical manifestations and morphological results of imaging studies. This helps better understand intracranial dynamics and activity of hydrocephalus in regard to indication and timing of drainage procedure.

Acknowledgements

This work was supported by a project on the application of PACS (Picture Archiving and Communication System) in the research and development, ITMS 26210120004.

Abbreviations

ACA	anterior cerebral artery
BA	basilar artery
ICA	internal carotid artery
ICP	intracranial pressure
ICV	internal cerebral vein
MCA	middle cerebral artery
ONSD	optic nerve sheath diameter
PI	pulsatility index
RI	resistance index
VA	vertebral artery
Ved	end-diastolic blood flow velocity
Vmean	mean blood flow velocity
Vsyst	maximal systolic blood flow velocity

Author details

Branislav Kolarovszki

Address all correspondence to: kolarovszki@jfmed.uniba.sk

Clinic of Neurosurgery, Jessenius Faculty of Medicine in Martin, Comenius University in Bratislava, University Hospital Martin, Martin, Slovakia

References

[1] Kolarovszki B, Zibolen M. Transcranial doppler ultrasonography in the management of neonatal hydrocephalus. In: Pant S, Cherian I, editors. Hydrocephalus. Rijeka: InTech; 2012. pp. 131-152

[2] Bada HS, Miller JE, Menke JA, Menten TG, Bashiru M, Binstadt D, Sumner DS, Khanna NN. Intracranial pressure and cerebral arterial pulsatile flow measurements in neonatal intraventricular haemorrhage. The Journal of Pediatrics. 1982;**100**:291-296

[3] Hill A, Volpe JJ. Decrease in pulsatile flow in anterior cerebral arteries in infantile hydrocephalus. Pediatrics. 1982;**69**:4-7

[4] Fisher AQ, Livingstone JN II. Transcranial Doppler and real-time cranial sonography in neonatal hydrocephalus. Journal of Child Neurology. 1989;**4**:64-69

[5] Aaslid R, Hubert P, Nornes H. Evaluation of cerebrovascular spasm with transcranial Doppler ultrasound. Journal of Neurosurgery. 1984;**60**:37-41

[6] De Assis MC, Machado HR. Transfontanellar Doppler ultrasound measurement of cerebral blood velocity before and after surgical treatment of hydrocephalus. Arquivos de Neuro-Psiquiatria. 1999;**57**(3B):827-835 abstract

[7] Nishimaki S, Yoda H, Seki K, Kawakami T, Akamatsu H, Iwasaki Y. Cerebral blood flow velocities in the anterior cerebral arteries and basilar artery in hydrocephalus before and after treatment. Surgical Neurology. 1990;**34**:373-377

[8] Sato O, Ohya M, Nojiri K, Tsugane R. Microcirculatory changes in experimental hydrocephalus: Morphological and physiological studies. In: Shapiro K, Marmarou A, Portnoy H, editors. Hydrocephalus. New York: Raven Press; 1984. pp. 215-230

[9] Nadvi SS, Du Trevou MD, Vandelen JR, Gouws E. The use of TCD ultrasonography as a method of assessing ICP in hydrocephalic children. British Journal of Neurosurgery. 1994; **8**:573-577

[10] Jindal A, Mahapatra AK. Correlation of ventricular size and transcranial Doppler findings before and after ventricular peritoneal shunt in patients with hydrocephalus: Prospective study of 35 patients. Journal of Neurology, Neurosurgery, and Psychiatry. 1998;**65**:269-271

[11] De Riggo J, Kolarovszki B, Richterová R, Kolarovszká H, Šutovský J, Ďurdík P. Measurement of the blood flow velocity in the pericallosal artery of children with hydrocephalus by transcranial Doppler ultrasonography—Preliminary results. Biomedical Papers. 2007; **151**:285-289

[12] Kolarovszki B, Žúbor P, Kolarovszká H, Benčo M, Richterová R, Maťašová K. The assessment of intracranial dynamics by transcranial Doppler sonography in perioperative period in paediatric hydrocephalus. Archives of Gynecology and Obstetrics. 2013;**287**:229-238

[13] Erol FS, Yakar H, Artas H, Kaplan M, Kaman D. Investigating a correlation between the results of transcranial Doppler and the level of nerve growth factor in cerebrospinal fluid of hydrocephalic infants: Clinical study. Pediatric Neurosurgery. 2009;**45**:192-197

[14] Uhríková Z, Kolarovszki B, Javorka K, Javorka M, Maťašová K, Kolarovszká H, Zibolen M. Changes in heart rate variability in a premature infant with hydrocephalus. American Journal of Perinatology Reports. 2012;**2**:43-46

[15] van Bel F, van de Bor M, Baan J, Stijnen T, Ruys JH. Blood flow velocity pattern of the anterior cerebral arteries. Journal of Ultrasound in Medicine. 1988;**7**:553-559

[16] Weller RO, Shulman K. Infantile hydrocephalus: Clinical, histological and ultrastructural study of brain damage. Journal of Neurosurgery. 1972;**36**:255-265

[17] Wozniak M, McLone DG, Raimondi AJ. Micro and macrovascular changes as a direct cause of parenchymal destruction in congenital murine hydrocephalus. Journal of Neurosurgery. 1975;**43**:535-545

[18] Alvisi C, Cerisoli M, Giulioni M, Monari P, Salvioli GP, Sandri F, Lippi C, Bovicelli L, Pilu G. Evaluation of cerebral blood flow changes by transfontanelle Doppler ultrasound in infantile hydrocephalus. Child's Nervous System. 1985;**1**:244-247

[19] Goh D, Minns RA, Pye SD, Steers AJ. Cerebral blood flow velocity changes after ventricular taps and ventriculoperitoneal shunting. Child's Nervous System. 1991;**7**:452-457

[20] Goh D, Minns RA, Hendry GM, Thambyayah M, Steers AJ. Cerebrovascular resistive index assessed by duplex Doppler sonography and its relationship to intracranial pressure in infantile hydrocephalus. Pediatric Radiology. 1992;**22**:246-250

[21] Iacopino DG, Zaccone C, Molina D, Todaro C, Tomasello F, Cardia E. Intraoperative monitoring of cerebral blood flow during ventricular shunting in hydrocephalic pediatric patients. Child's Nervous System. 1995;**11**:483-486

[22] Cosan TE, Gucuyener D, Dundar E, Arslantas A, Vural M, Uzuner K, Tel E. Cerebral blood flow alterations in progressive communicating hydrocephalus: Transcranial Doppler assessment in an experimental model. Neurosurgical Focus. 2000;**9**:1-5

[23] Del Bigio MR. Neuropathological changes caused by hydrocephalus. Acta Neuropathologica. 1993;**85**:573-585

[24] Quinn MW, Pople IK. MCA pulsatility in children with blocked CSF shunt. Journal of Neurology, Neurosurgery, and Psychiatry. 1992;**55**:525-527

[25] Goh D, Minns RA. Intracranial pressure and cerebral arterial flow velocity indices in childhood hydrocephalus: Current review. Child's Nervous System. 1995;**11**:392-396

[26] Finn JP, Quinn MW, Hall-Craggs MA, Kendall BE. Impact of vessel distortion on transcranial Doppler velocity measurements: Correlation with magnetic resonance imaging. Journal of Neurosurgery. 1990;**73**:572-575

[27] Volpe JJ. Neurology of the newborn. 4th ed. Vol. 2001. Philadelphia: WB Saunders; 2001. p. 428

[28] Anca IA. Hypoxic ischemic cerebral lesions of the newborn—Ultrasound diagnosis. Pictorial essay. Medical Ultrasonography. 2011;**13**:314-319

[29] Schellinger D, Grant EG, Richardson JD. Cystic periventricular leukomalacia: Sonographic and CT findings. American Journal of Neuroradiology. 1984;**5**:439-445

[30] Tsuji M, Saul JP, du Plessis A, Eichenwald E, Sobh J, Crocker R, Volpe JJ. Cerebral intravascular oxygenation correlates with mean arterial pressure in critically ill premature infants. Pediatrics. 2000;**106**:625-632

[31] Fukuda S, Kato T, Kakita H, Yamada Y, Hussein HM, Kato I, Suzuki S, Togari H. Hemodynamics of the cerebral arteries of infants with periventricular leukomalatia. Pediatrics. 2006;**117**:1-8

[32] Fukuda S, Mizuno K, Kakita H, Kato T, Hussein MH, Ito T, Daoud GA, Kato I, Suzuki S, Togari H. Late circulatory dysfunction and decreased cerebral blood flow volume in infants with periventricular leukomalacia. Brain and Development. 2008;**30**:589-594

[33] Ilves P, Lintrop M, Talvik I, Muug K, Maipuu L, Metsvaht T. Low cerebral blood flow velocity and head circumference in infants with severe hypoxic ischemic encephalopathy and poor outcome. Acta Paediatrica. 2009;**98**:459-465

[34] Liu J, Cao HY, Huang XH, Wang Q. The pattern and early diagnostic value of Doppler ultrasound for neonatal hypoxic-ischemic encephalopathy. Journal of Tropical Pediatrics. 2007;**53**:351-354

[35] Papile L, Burnstein J, Burnstein R, Koffler H. Incidence and evolution of subependymal and intraventricular hemorrhage: A study of infants with birth weights less than 1,500 gm. The Journal of Pediatrics. 1978;**92**:529-534

[36] Taylor GA, Madsen JR. Neonatal hydrocephalus: Hemodynamic response to fontanelle compression—correlation with intracranial pressure and need for shunt placement. Radiology. 1996;**201**:685-689

[37] McCrea HJ, Ment LR. The diagnosis, management, and postnatal prevention of intraventricular hemorrhage in the preterm neonate. Clinics in Perinatology. 2008;**35**:777-792

[38] Miranda P. Intraventricular hemorrhage and posthemorrhagic hydrocephalus in the preterm infant. Minerva Pediatrica. 2010;**62**:79-89

[39] Tsitouras V, Sgouros S. Infantile posthemorrhagic hydrocephalus. Child's Nervous System. 2011;**27**:1595-1608

[40] Bada HS, Hajjar W, Chua C, Summer DS. Noninvasive diagnosis of neonatal asphyxia and intraventricular hemorrhage by Doppler ultrasound. The Journal of Pediatrics. 1979;**95**: 775-779

[41] Bashiru M, Russell J, Bada HS, Menke JA, Miles R, Summer D. Noninvasive detection of neonatal cerebrovascular disease. Bruit. 1980;**4**:42

[42] Ventriculomegaly Trial Group. Randomised trial of early tapping in neonatal posthaemorrhagic ventricular dilatation. Archives of Disease in Childhood;**65**:3-10

[43] Nishimaki S, Iwasaki Y, Akamatsu H. Cerebral blood flow velocity before and after cerebrospinal fluid drainage in infants with posthemorrhagic hydrocephalus. Journal of Ultrasound in Medicine. 2004;**23**:1315-1319

[44] Kempley ST, Gamsu HR. Changes in cerebral artery blood flow velocity after intermittent cerebrospinal fluid drainage. Archives of Disease in Childhood. 1993;**63**:74-76

[45] Quinn MW, Ando Y, Levene MI. Cerebral arterial and venous flow-velocity measurements in post-haemorrhagic ventricular dilatation and hydrocephalus. Developmental Medicine and Child Neurology. 1992;**34**:863-869

[46] Maertzdorf WJ, Vles JS, Beuls E, Mulder ALM, Blanco CE. Intracranial pressure and cerebral blood flow velocity in preterm infants with posthaemorrhagic ventricular dilatation. Archives of Disease in Childhood. Fetal and Neonatal Edition. 2002;**87**:185-188

[47] Soul JS, Eichenwald E, Walter G, Volpe JJ, du Plessis AJ. CSF removal in infantile posthemorrhagic hydrocephalus results in significant improvement in cerebral hemodynamics. Pediatric Research. 2004;**55**:872-876

[48] van Alfen-van der Velden AA, Hopman JC, Klaessens JH, Feuth T, Sengers RC, Liem KD. Cerebral hemodynamics and oxygenation after serial CSF drainage in infants with PHVD. Brain and Development. 2007;**29**:623-629

[49] Pople IK. Doppler flow velocities in children with controlled hydrocephalus: Reference values for the diagnosis of blocked cerebrospinal fluid shunts. Child's Nervous System. 1992;**8**:124-125

[50] Pople IK, Quinn MW, Bayston R, Hayward RD. The Doppler pulsatility index as a screening test for blocked ventriculo-peritoneal shunts. European Journal of Pediatric Surgery. 1991;**1**(Suppl):27-29

[51] Chadduck WM, Crabtree HM, Blankenship JB, Adametz J. Transcranial Doppler ultrasonography for the evaluation of shunt malfunction in pediatric patients. Child's Nervous System. 1991;**7**:27-30

[52] Vajda Z, Büki A, Vető F, Horváth Z, Sándor J, Dóczi T. Transcranial Doppler-determined pulsatility index in the evaluation of endoscopic third ventriculostomy (preliminary data). Acta Neurochirurgica. 1999;**141**:247-250

[53] De Oliveira RS, Machado HR. Transcranial color-coded Doppler ultrasonography for evaluation of children with hydrocephalus. Neurosurgical Focus. 2003;**15**:1-7

[54] Taylor GA, Phillips MD, Ichord RN, Carson BS, Gates JA, James CS. Intracranial compliance in infants: Evaluation with Doppler US. Radiology. 1994;**191**:787-791

[55] Westra SJ, Lazareff J, Curran JG, Sayere JW, Kawamoto H Jr. Transcranial Doppler ultrasonography to evaluate need for cerebrospinal fluid drainage in hydrocephalic children. Journal of Ultrasound in Medicine. 1998;**17**:561-569

[56] Gera P, Gupta R, Sailukar M, Agarwal P, Parelkar S, Oak S. Role of transcranial Doppler sonography and pressure provacation test to evaluate the need for cerebrospinal fluid drainage in hydrocephalic children. Journal of Indian Association of Pediatric Surgeons. 2002;**7**:174-183

[57] Taylor GA. Effect of scanning pressure on the intracranial hemodynamics during transfontanellar duplex Doppler examinations. Radiology. 1992;**185**:763-766

[58] Behrens A, Lenfeldt N, Ambarki K, Malm J, Eklund A, Koskinen LO. Transcranial Doppler pulsatility index: Not an accurate method to assess intracranial pressure. Neurosurgery. 2010;**66**:1050-1057

[59] Hanlo PW, Gooskens RH, Nijhuis IJ, Faber JA, Peters RJ, van Huffelen AC, Tulleken CA, Willemse J. Value of transcranial Doppler indices in predicting raised ICP in infantile hydrocephalus. A study with review of literature. Child's Nervous System. 1995;**11**:595-603

[60] Hanlo PW, Peters RJ, Gooskens RH, Heethaar RM, Keunen RW, van Huffelen AC, Tulleken CA, Willemse J. Monitoring intracranial dynamics by transcranial Doppler—A new Doppler index: Trans systolic time. Ultrasound in Medicine & Biology. 1995;**21**:613-621

[61] Leliefeld PH, Gooskens RH, Peters RJ, Tulleken CA, Kappelle LJ, Han KS, Regli L, Hanlo PW. New transcranial Doppler index in infants with hydrocephalus: Transsystolic time in clinical practice. Ultrasound in Medicine & Biology. 2009;**35**:1601-1606

[62] Leliefeld PH, Gooskens RH, Tulleken CA, Regli L, Uiterwaal CS, Han KS, Kappelle LJ. Noninvasive detection of the distinction between progressive and compensated hydrocephalus in infants: Is it possible ? Journal of Neurosurgery. Pediatrics. 2010;**5**:562-568

[63] Galarza M, Lazareff JA. Transcranial Doppler in infantile cerebrospinal fluid disorders: Clinical validity. Neurological Research. 2004;**26**:409-413

[64] Rodríguez-Nuñez A, Somoza-Martín M, Gómez-Lado C, Eirís-Puñal J, Camiña-Darriba F, Rodríguez-Segade S, Castro-Gago M. Therapeutic criteria in communicating childhood hydrocephalus. Journal of Neurosurgical Sciences. 2008;**52**:17-21

[65] Liu D, Li Z, Zhang X, Zhao L, Jia J, Sun F, Wang Y, Ma D, Wei W. Assessment of intracranial pressure with ultrasonographic retrobulbar optic nerve sheath diameter measurement. BMC Neurology. 2017;**17**(1):188

[66] Maissan IM, Dirven PJ, Haitsma IK, Hoeks SE, Gommers D, Stolker RJ. Ultrasonographic measured optic nerve sheath diameter as an accurate and quick monitor for changes in intracranial pressure. Journal of Neurosurgery. 2015;**123**(3):743-747

[67] Messerer M, Berhouma M, Messerer R, Dubourg J. Interest of optic nerve sheath diameter ultrasonography in detecting non-invasively raised intracranial pressure. Neuro-Chirurgie. 2013;**59**(2):55-59

[68] Soldatos T, Chatzimichail K, Papathanasiou M, Gouliamos A. Optic nerve sonography: A new window for the non-invasive evaluation of intracranial pressure in brain injury. Emergency Medicine Journal. 2009;**26**(9):630-634

[69] Ragauskas A, Bartusis L, Piper I, Zakelis R, Matijosaitis V, Petrikonis K, Rastenyte D. Improved diagnostic value of a TCD-based non-invasive ICP measurement method compared with the sonographic ONSD method for detecting elevated intracranial pressure. Neurological Research. 2014;**36**(7):607-614

[70] Tarzamni MK, Derakhshan B, Meshkini A, Merat H, Fouladi DF, Mostafazadeh S, Rezakhah A. The diagnostic performance of ultrasonographic optic nerve sheath diameter and color Doppler indices of the ophthalmic arteries in detecting elevated intracranial pressure. Clinical Neurology and Neurosurgery. 2016;**141**:82-88

Chapter 5

3D Numerical Study of Metastatic Tumor Blood Perfusion and Interstitial Fluid Flow Based on Microvasculature Response to Inhibitory Effect of Angiostatin

Gaiping Zhao

Additional information is available at the end of the chapter

http://dx.doi.org/10.5772/intechopen.78949

Abstract

Metastatic tumor blood perfusion and interstitial fluid transport based on 3D microvasculature response to inhibitory effect of angiostatin are investigated. 3D blood flow, interstitial fluid transport, and transvascular flow are described by the extended Poiseuille's, Darcy's, and Starling's law, respectively. The simulation results demonstrate that angiostatin has the capacity to regulate and inhibit the formation of new blood vessels and has an obvious impact on the morphology, growth rate, and the branches of microvascular network inside and outside the metastatic tumor. Heterogeneous blood perfusion, widespread interstitial hypertension, and low convection within the metastatic tumor have obviously improved under the inhibitory effect of angiostatin, which suits well with the experimental observations. They can also result in more efficient drug delivery and penetration into the metastatic tumor. The simulation results may provide beneficial information and theoretical models for clinical research of antiangiogenic therapy strategies.

Keywords: blood perfusion, interstitial transport, metastatic tumor, angiostatin, 3D simulation

1. Introduction

Cancer is the second leading cause of mortality worldwide [1], right behind cardiovascular disease. Metastatic tumors, the ultimate causes of death for the majority of cancer patients, are the important biological characteristics of malignant tumors. Metastasis occurs when cancer

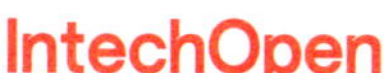

cells spread from a primary tumor to distant and vital organs (secondary sites) in human body. Angiogenesis is necessary for tumor growth, invasion, and metastasis [2], since it supplies the nutrients and oxygen for continued tumor growth. The neovascularization accelerates the growth of tumor while simultaneously offering an initial route by which cancer cells can escape from a primary tumor to form metastatic tumor. Cancer cells migrate into the blood stream and surrounding tissues via microcirculation, then continue to grow giving rise to metastases [3]. The blood perfusion and interstitial fluid flow have been recognized as critical elements in metastatic tumor growth and vascularization [4]. However, tumor vessels are dilated, saccular, tortuous, and heterogeneous in their spatial distribution. These abnormalities result in heterogeneity of blood flow and elevated interstitial fluid pressure (IFP), which forms a physiological barrier to the delivery of therapeutic agents to tumors [5]. Abnormal microvasculature and microenvironment further lowers the effectiveness of therapeutic agents.

Experimental research showed that the primary tumor in the Lewis lung model system was capable of generating a factor which was named angiostatin later suppressing the neovascularization and expansion of tumor metastases [6]. Angiostatin is a 38-kD internal peptide of plasminogen, which is a potent inhibitor of angiogenesis in vivo, and selectively inhibits endothelial cell (EC) proliferation and migration in vitro. Tumor cells express enzymatic activity which is capable of hydrolyzing plasminogen to generate angiostatin [7]. Angiostatin is then transported and accumulated in the blood circulation in excess of the stimulators and thus inhibiting angiogenesis of a metastatic tumor. Angiostatin, by virtue of its longer half-life in the circulation [8], reaches the vascular bed of metastatic tumor. As a result, growth of a metastasis is restricted by preventing and inhibiting angiogenesis within the vascular bed of the metastasis itself. A schematic diagram of this process is given in **Figure 1**. Indeed, anti-angiogenic treatments directly targeting angiogenic signaling pathways as well as indirectly modulating angiogenesis show normalization of tumor microvasculature and microenvironment at least transiently in both preclinical and clinical settings.

In spite of several mathematical models of metastatic tumors, there appears to be little in the literature by way of mathematical modeling of the mechanisms of antiangiogenic activity of angiostatin on blood flow and interstitial fluid pressure in a metastatic tumor. Liotta et al. [9] first

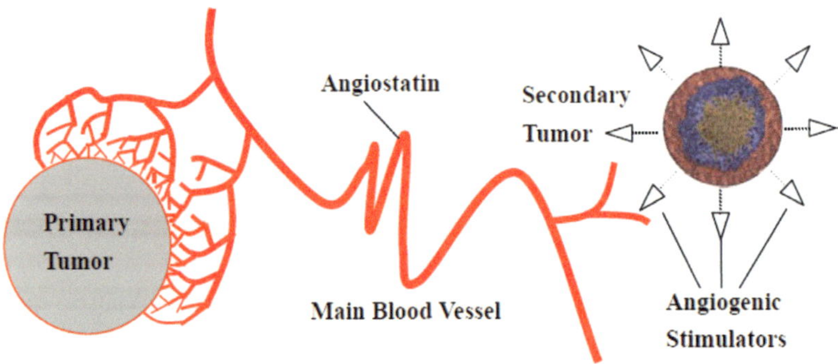

Figure 1. Schematic representation of angiostatin transported from a fully vascularized primary tumor to its relation to a distant secondary tumor.

developed an experimental model to quantify some of the major processes initiated by tumor transplantation and culminating in pulmonary metastases. The study suggested that "dynamics of hematogenously initiated metastases depended strongly on the entry rate of tumor cell clumps into the circulation, which in turn was intimately linked to tumor vascularization." Later in the study, Liotta et al. [9] confirmed their former observation and raised the idea that "larger clumps produce significantly more metastatic foci than do smaller clumps matched for the number of cells." Saidel et al. [10] proposed a lumped-parameter, deterministic model of the hematogenous metastatic process from a solid tumor, which provided a general theoretical framework for analysis and simulation. Numerical solutions of the model were in good agreement with their experimental results [9]. The possibilities of anti-invasion and antimetastatic strategies in cancer treatment have bestowed an added preponderance with the keen interest in the mathematical modeling in the areas of tumor invasion and metastasis. Orme and Chaplain [11] presented a simple mathematical model of the vascularization and subsequent growth of a solid spherical tumor and gave a possible explanation for tumor metastasis, whereby tumor cells entered the blood system and secondary tumor may rise with the transportation function of blood. Sleeman and Nimmo [12] modified the model of fluid transport in vascularized tumors by Baxter and Jain [13] to take tumor invasion and metastasis into consideration. Although these models did provide some features of tumor metastasis and interstitial fluid transportation such as perturbation analysis, they lacked in providing more detail information of metastatic tumor and as such were of limited predicted value. More realistic models of metastasis and interstitial fluid transportation were developed to better understand its mechanism. Anderson et al. [14] presented a discrete model from the partial differential equations of the continuum models which implied that haptotaxis was important for tumor metastasis. Iwata et al. [15] proposed a partial differential equation (PDE) that described the metastatic evolution of an untreated tumor, and its predicted results agreed well with successive data of a clinically observed metastatic tumor. Benzekry et al. [16] proposed an organism-scale model for the development of a population of secondary tumors that takes into account systemic inhibiting interactions among tumors due to the release of a circulating angiogenesis inhibitor. Baratchart et al. [17] derived a mathematical model of spatial tumor growth compared with experimental data and suggested that the dynamics of metastasis relied on spatial interactions between metastatic lesions. Stéphanou et al. [18] investigated chemotherapy treatment efficiency by performing a Newtonian fluid flow simulation based on a study of vascular networks generated from a mathematical model of tumor angiogenesis. Wu et al. [19] extended the mathematical model into a 3D case to investigate tumor blood perfusion and interstitial fluid movements originating from tumor-induced angiogenesis. Soltani and Chen [20] first studied the fluid flow in a tumor-induced capillary network and the interstitial fluid flow in normal and tumor tissues. The model provided a more realistic prediction of interstitial fluid flow pattern in solid tumor than the previous models. Some related works have been done on tumor-induced angiogenesis, blood perfusion, and interstitial fluid flow in the tumor microenvironment by using 2D mathematical methods [5, 21–23]. In spite of the valuable body of work performed in simulation of blood perfusion, interstitial fluid flow, and metastasis, previous studies have not examined blood perfusion and interstitial fluid pressure in the metastatic tumor microcirculation based on the 3D microvascular network response to the inhibitory effect of angiostatin which plays a significant role in suppressing tumor growth and metastasis.

Metastatic tumor blood perfusion and interstitial fluid transport based on 3D microvasculature response to inhibitory effect of angiostatin are investigated for exploring the suppression of metastatic tumor growth by the primary tumor. The abnormal geometric and morphological features of 3D microvasculature network inside and outside the metastatic tumor, and relative complex and heterogeneous hemodynamic characteristics in the presence and absence of angiostatin can be studied in the 3D case. The simulation results may provide beneficial information and theoretical basis for clinical research on antiangiogenic therapy.

2. 3D mathematical models

2.1. Metastatic tumor angiogenesis

3D mathematical model we present in this section originates from the previous 2D tumor antiangiogenesis mathematical model [5, 21] describing how capillary networks form in a metastatic tumor in response to angiostatin released by a primary tumor. The conservation equation of endothelial cells (EC) indicates the migration of EC influenced mainly by four factors: random motility, inhibitory effect of angiostatin, chemotaxis, and haptotaxis. Subsequently, from a discretized form of the partial differential equations governing endothelial-cell motion, a discrete biased random-walk model will be derived enabling the paths of individual endothelial cells located at the sprout tips, and hence the individual capillary sprouts, to be followed. Hence, realistic capillary network structures were generated by incorporating rules for sprout branching and anastomosis. The generated microvascular network inside and outside the metastatic tumor in the presence of angiostatin and in the absence of angiostatin is shown in **Figure 2**. General morphological features of the network such as growth speed, capillary number, vessel branching order, and anastomosis density in/outside the metastatic tumor are consistent with the physiologically observed results, which indicate that angiostatin secreted by the primary tumor dose has an inhibitory effect on metastatic tumor [5, 11].

2.2. Blood perfusion

To calculate blood flow through a given 3D microvascular network of interconnected capillary elements to the metastatic tumor, assuming flux conservation and incompressible flow at each junction where the capillary elements meet

$$\sum_{n=1}^{6} Q^n_{(l.m.j)} \cdot B^n_{(l.m,j)} = 0 \tag{1}$$

where $B^n_{(l,m,j)}$ takes the integer 1 or 0, representing the connectivity between node (l, m, j) and its adjacent node n. $Q^n_{(l,m,j)}$ is the flow rate from node (l, m, j) to node n and is given by $Q^n_{(l.m.j)} = Q^n_{v,(l,m,j)} - Q^n_{t,(l,m,j)}$, where $Q^n_{v,(l,m,j)}$ is the vascular flow rate without fluid leakage, described locally by Poiseuille's law

$$Q^n_{v,(l.m,j)} = \frac{\pi R^4_n (p_{v,(l,m,j)} - p_{v,(n)})}{8\,\mu_n\,\Delta L_n} \tag{2}$$

and $Q^n_{t,(l,m,j)}$ is the transvascular flow rate, following Starling's law

http://dx.doi.org/10.5772/intechopen.78949

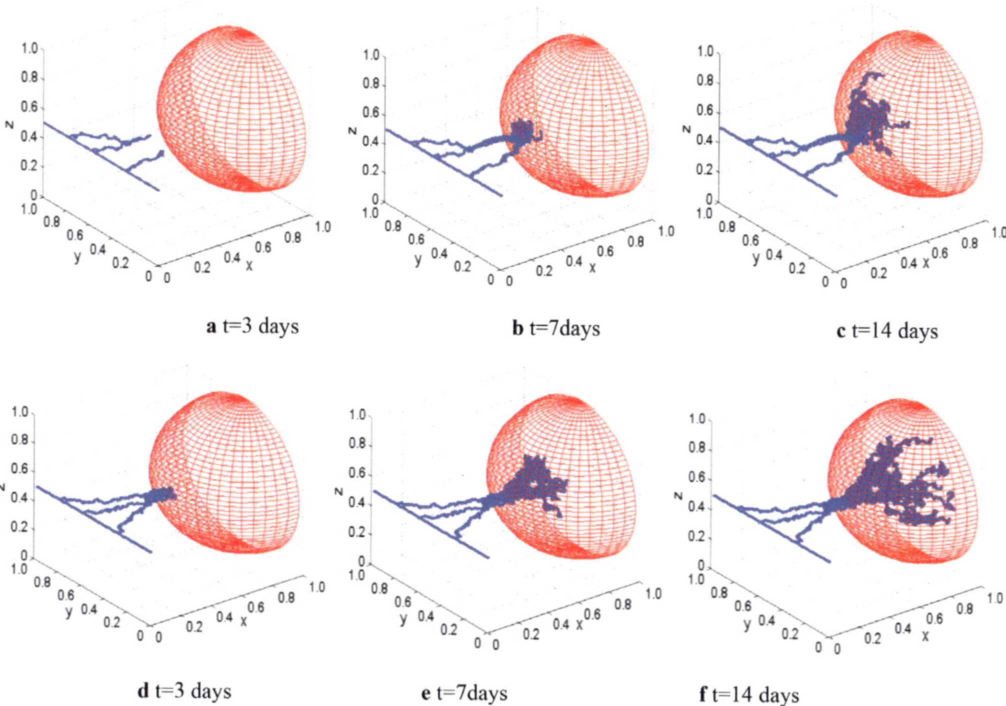

Figure 2. The spatiotemporal dynamic growth of 3D microvascular networks inside and outside the metastatic tumor: (a–c) in the presence of angiostatin; (d–f) in the absence of angiostatin.

$$Q^n_{t,(l,m,j)} = 2\pi R_n \Delta L_n \cdot L_{pv}\left[\left(\bar{p}^n_{v,(l,m,j)} - \bar{p}^n_{i,(l,m,j)}\right) - \sigma_t(\pi_v - \pi_i)\right] \tag{3}$$

where $p_{v,(l,m,j)}$ and $p_{v,(n)}$ are the intravascular pressure of node (l, m, j) and node n; $\bar{p}^n_{v,(l,m,j)}$ is the mean pressure in vascular element (l, m, j); $\bar{p}^n_{i,(l,m,j)}$ is the mean interstitial pressure outside of vascular element (l, m, j). μ_n, R_n, and ΔL_n are the blood viscosity, radius, and length of the vessel element n, respectively; L_{pv} is the hydraulic permeability of vascular wall; σ_t is the average osmotic reflection coefficient for plasma proteins; π_v and π_i are the colloid osmotic pressure of plasma and interstitial fluid.

2.3. Interstitial flow in metastatic tumor

Considering the metastatic tumor tissue as an isotropic porous medium, its interstitial flow is modeled by Darcy's law [24]:

$$\boldsymbol{u}_i = -\kappa \nabla p_i \tag{4}$$

where $\boldsymbol{u}_i$ is the interstitial fluid velocity; κ is the hydraulic conductivity coefficient of the interstitium; p_i is the interstitial pressure.

The continuity equation is given by:

$$\nabla \cdot \boldsymbol{u}_i = \phi_v - \phi_L \tag{5}$$

where $\phi_v = \frac{L_{pv} S_v}{V}(p_v - p_i - \sigma_t(\pi_v - \pi_i))$ is the fluid source term leaking from blood vessels. $\phi_L = \frac{L_{pL} S_L}{V}(p_i - p_L)$ is the lymphatic drainage term, which is proportional to the pressure difference between the interstitium and the lymphatics.

Mass conservation at each junction where the interstitial fluid pressure satisfies equation:

$$\nabla^2 p_i = \frac{\alpha^2}{R^2}(p_i - p_{ev}) \cdot B \tag{6}$$

where $p_{ev} = (L_{pv} S_v(p_v - \sigma_t(\pi_v - \pi_i)) + L_{pL} S_L p_L)/(L_{pv} S_v + L_{pL} S_L)$ is the effective pressure and $\alpha = R\sqrt{(L_{pv} S_v + L_{pL} S_L)/\kappa V}$ is the ratio of interstitial to vascular resistances to fluid flow. L_{pL} is the hydraulic permeability of lymphatic vessel wall. S_v/V and S_L/V are the surface areas of blood vessel wall and lymphatic vessel wall per unit volume of tissue. In the model, $L_{pL} S_L/V$ is assumed zero for tumor tissue, and given a uniform value for normal tissue referring to Baxter and Jain [13]. The continuity of pressure and flux on the interconnected boundary between the tumor and normal tissue Γ: $p_i|_{\Gamma^-} = p_i|_{\Gamma^+}, -\kappa_T \nabla p_i|_{\Gamma^-} = -\kappa_N \nabla p_i|_{\Gamma^+}$, κ_T, and κ_N are the hydraulic conductivity coefficients of normal tissue and tumor tissue, respectively.

Table 1 shows the values of the parameters used in the microcirculation simulations.

Parameter	Name	Value	Parameter	Name	Value
σ_t^{a}	Average osmotic reflection coefficient for plasma proteins	$8.7 \times 10^{-5}{}_{T}$ 091_{N}	κ^{a}	Hydraulic conductivity coefficient of interstitium	$2.5 \times 10^{-7}{}_{T}$ cm²/mmHg s $2.5 \times 10^{-7}{}_{N}$ cm²/mmHg s
π_v^{a}	Colloid osmotic pressure of plasma	198_T mmHg 20_N mmHg	$\left(\frac{S_v}{V}\right)^{a}$	Surface area per unit volume for transport in interstitium	50_T cm^{-1} 50_N cm^{-1}
p_L^{c}	Lymphatic pressure	0.5_N mmHg	$\frac{L_{pL} S_L}{V}^{c}$	Absorption capacity of lymphatic system	0_T 1/mmHg s $1.0 \times 10^{-4}{}_{N}$ 1/mmHg s
π_i^{a}	Colloid osmotic pressure of interstitium	173_T mmHg 10_N mmHg	L_{pv}^{a}	Hydraulic permeability of vascular wall	$1.86 \times 10^{-6}{}_{T}$ cm/mmHg s $3.6 \times 10^{-8}{}_{N}$ cm/mmHg s
μ^{b}	Blood viscosity	1.0 cP			

[a]Jain et al. [5].

[b]Stephanou et al. [18].

[c]Zhao et al. [25].

Subscript "N" and "T" represents the values in normal and tumor tissues, respectively.

Table 1. Baseline parameter values used in the simulations.

3. Simulation results

3.1. 3D blood perfusion of metastatic tumor

We simulated the evolution of blood flow pressure in the presence/absence of angiostatin for 14 days representing the typical timescale for tumor vasculature to grow. **Figure 3** shows

http://dx.doi.org/10.5772/intechopen.78949

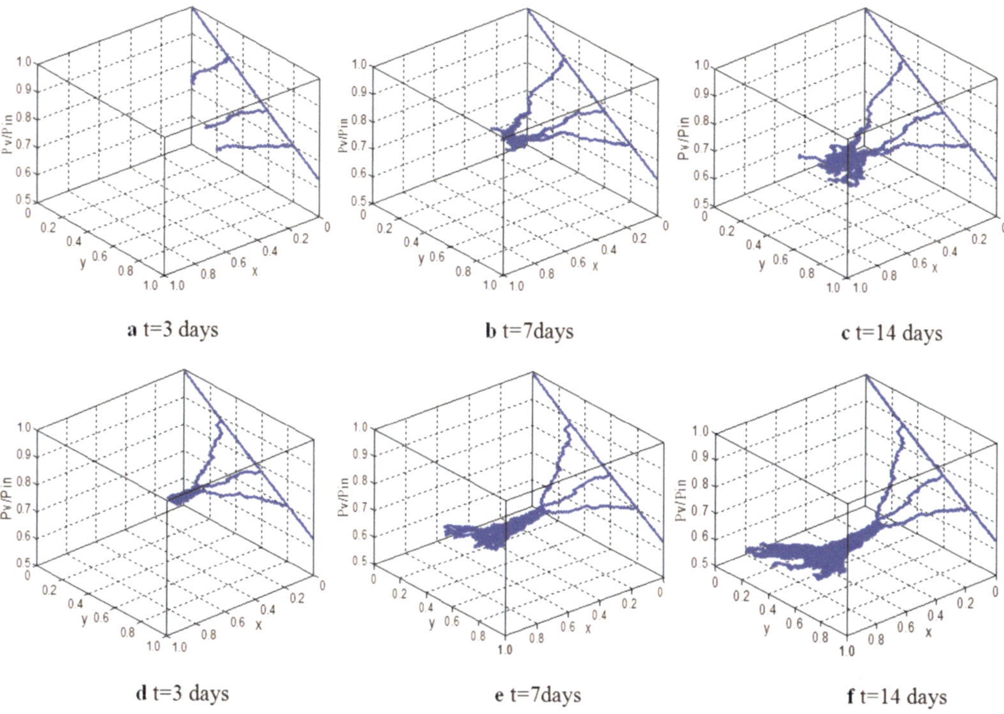

Figure 3. Simulations of blood pressure through 3D microvascular networks over time: (a–c) example simulation with angiostatin; (d–f) example simulation without angiostatin. Simulation domain is $[0, 1] \times [0, 1] \times [0, 1]$. Blood enters the networks at the end of the parent vessel ($x = 0, y = 0, z = 0.5$), distributes throughout the capillary network, leaves from the end of the parent vessel ($x = 0, y = 1, z = 0.5$).

the snapshots of the pressure profiles of blood flow through each vessel segment in a three-dimensional microvascular networks. We keep the inlet pressure and outlet pressure across parent vessel fixed at 25 and 16 mmHg [25] in the simulation, in accordance with physiological values at the capillary scale. **Figure 3** highlights a direct comparison of blood pressure distributions (**Figure 3a–c** shows the blood pressure distribution in the presence of angiostatin, **Figure 3d–f** shows the blood pressure distribution in the absence of angiostatin). We observe that the overall blood pressure is higher in the presence of angiostatin than that in the absence of angiostatin over the same growth duration. The blood flow distribution is complex and chaotic which makes the variety of blood pressure small in the interior of the metastatic tumor compared to its exterior, contributing to the difficulties of efficient drug delivery in metastatic tumor. In the presence of angiostatin, the pressure-flows within some of the daughter vessels are elevated from the branching points to the metastatic tumor surface which provides effective blood perfusion and thus efficient therapeutic agents to the tumor. The simulation results indicate that blood perfusion varies significantly with the complex and chaotic three-dimensional microvascular networks inside and outside the metastatic tumor. The poor blood perfusion can be improved through the increased intravascular pressure with the presence of angiostatin. These results suggest that the inhibitory effect of angiostatin can affect the distribution of blood flow pressure and improve drug delivery to tumor.

3.2. 3D interstitial fluid flow of metastatic tumor

Figure 4 shows the distribution of interstitial fluid pressure (IFP) within the metastatic tumor under the two mentioned situations. From the simulation results, we obtain that maximum IFP near the tumor center significantly dropped from 3.3, 11.48, and 11.53 to 0, 4.7, and 10.3 mmHg

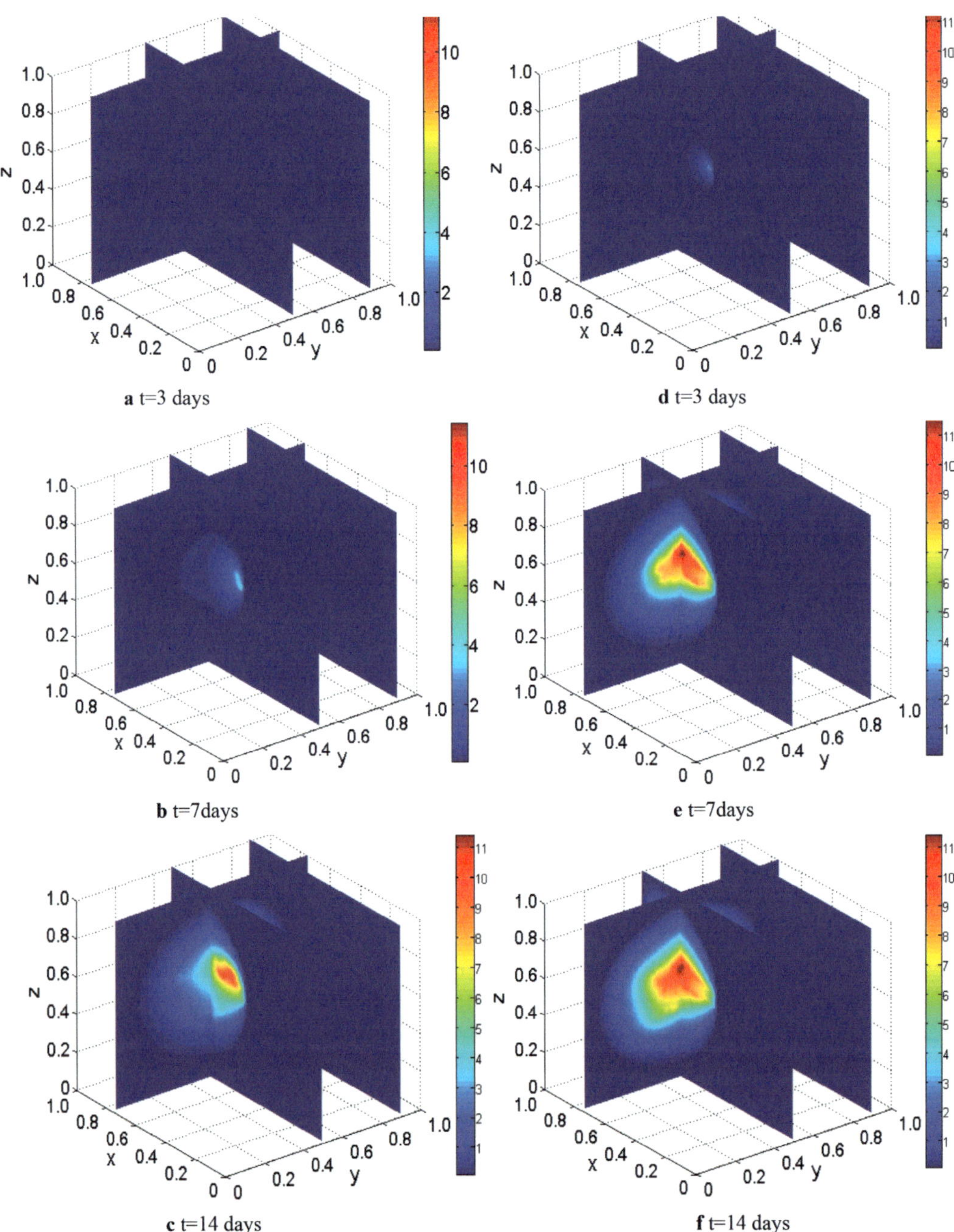

a t=3 days

d t=3 days

b t=7days

e t=7days

c t=14 days

f t=14 days

Figure 4. Interstitial fluid pressure distributions within the metastatic tumor: (a–c) in the presence of angiostatin; (d–f) in the absence of angiostatin on the same other conditions.

http://dx.doi.org/10.5772/intechopen.78949

with the presence of angiostatin at t = 3, 7 and 14 days, respectively, which indicated the IFP plateau is well relieved. As the growth days increase, IFP gradually elevates throughout the 3D metastatic tumor and the high pressure zone is at the center of the tumor and diminishes to the periphery and later becomes flatter. Comparing **Figure 4a–c** to **Figure 4d–f**, we come to conclude that angiostatin decreases the high IFP in the tumor, thus with the lower transvascular pressure in the 3D heterogeneous capillary networks, leading to an significantly improved situation for interstitial convection which plays a significant role in nonuniform distribution of drug delivery to the metastatic tumor. These results provide important references for cancer prevention and treatment. Furthermore, antiangiogenic therapies can normalize tumor vasculature and microenvironment, at least transiently in both preclinical and clinical settings [5].

4. Conclusion

The inhibitory effect of angiostatin on the growth of metastatic tumor has been observed in some clinical and experimental malignancies. In this chapter, we develop three-dimensional mathematical models describing the metastatic tumor microvasculature and microenvironment to investigate the inhibitory effect of antiangiogenic factor angiostatin secreted by the primary tumor on metastatic tumor angiogenesis, blood perfusion, and interstitial fluid flow. Simulation results demonstrate that angiostatin has an obvious impact on the morphology, expansion speed, capillary number, and vessel branching order inside and outside the metastatic tumor. 2D and 3D mathematical models of tumor antiangiogenesis predict similar morphological behavior, such as vessels' length, branching patterns, anastomosis density, or geometric distribution, for metastatic tumor angiogenesis under the inhibitory efficiency of angiostatin. However, capillary number and microvascular density due to space growth of vessel networks are increased in the 3D model. Furthermore, the simulations reflect the influences of heterogeneous blood perfusion, widespread interstitial hypertension, and low convection within the 3D metastatic tumor by carrying out a comparative study relating to the inhibitory effect of angiostatin. We find that 2D antiangiogenesis model may be well suited to studying morphological behavior of vessel networks in the metastatic tumor, but 3D antiangiogenesis model can better analyze blood perfusion, interstitial fluid flow, or oxygen and nutrient transport within the metastatic tumor microenvironment based on its more realistic 3D microvascular networks. Although 3D simulation results are consistent with the experimental observed facts and can provide more detailed space information, however, angiogenesis and hemodynamics in the metastatic tumor by the antiangiogenic therapy are very complex. To further research tumor angiogenic mechanisms and help to improve antiangiogenic cancer therapy, more realistic features and complex biology factors need to be incorporated within the 3D model, such as the anatomy and physiology of the metastatic tumor, drug delivery of antiangiogenic therapy, behaviors of cells adhesion and interaction and coupled with the various factors or other therapy strategies.

Acknowledgements

This research is supported by the National Natural Science Foundation of China (No. 11502146), Shanghai Natural Science Foundation (No. 15ZR1429600).

Conflict of interest

The authors declare that there is no conflict of interest regarding the publication of this chapter.

Author details

Gaiping Zhao

Address all correspondence to: zgp_06@126.com

School of Medical Instrument and Food Engineering, University of Shanghai for Science and Technology, Shanghai, China

References

[1] Siegel R, Naishadham D, Jemal A. Cancer statistics 2013. CA: A Cancer Journal for Clinicians. 2013;**63**:11e30

[2] Folkman J. Tumor angiogenesis: Therapeutic implications. New England Journal of Medicine. 1971;**285**(10):1182-1186

[3] Konjevi G, Stankovi S. Matrix metalloproteinases in the process of invasion and metastasis of breast cancer. Archive of Oncology. 2006;**14**(3-4):136-140

[4] Heldin CH, Rubin K, Pietras K, Ostman A. High interstitial fluid pressure—An obstacle in cancer therapy. Nature Reviews Cancer. 2004;**4**(10):806-813

[5] Jain RK, Tong RT, Munn LL. Effect of vascular normalization by antiangiogenic therapy on interstitial hypertension, peritumor edema, and lymphatic metastasis: Insights from a mathematical model. Cancer Research. 2007;**67**(6):2729-2735

[6] O'Reilly MS, Holmgren L, Shing Y, Chen C, Rosenthal RA, Moses M, Lane WS, Cao YH, Sage EH, Folkman J. Angiostatin: A novel angiogenesis inhibitor that mediates the suppression of metastases by a Lewis lung carcinoma. Cell. 1994;**79**:315-328

[7] Sim BKL, O'Reilly MS, Liang H, Fortier AH, He W, Madsen JW, Lapcevich R, Nancy CA. A recombinant human angiostatin protein inhibits experimental primary and metastatic cancer. Cancer Research. 1997;**57**(7):1329-1334

[8] Paweletz N, Knierim M. Tumor-related angiogenesis. Critical Reviews in Oncology/Hematology. 1989;**9**(3):197-242

[9] Liotta LA, Kleinerman J, Saidel GM. Quantitative relationships of intravascular tumor cells, tumor vessels, and pulmonary metastases following tumor implantation. Cancer Research. 1974;**34**(5):997-1004

[10] Saidel GM, Liotta LA, Kleinerman J. System dynamics of a metastatic process from an implanted tumor. Journal of Theoretical Biology. 1976;**56**(2):417-434

[11] Orme ME, Chaplain MAJ. A mathematical model of vascular tumour growth and invasion. Mathematical and Computer Modelling. 1996;**23**(10):43-60

[12] Sleeman BD, Nimmo HR. Fluid transport in vascularized tumours and metastasis. IMA Journal of Mathematics Applied in Medicine and Biology. 1998;**15**(1):53

[13] Baxter LT, Jain RK. Transport of fluid and macromolecules in tumors. I. Role of interstitial pressure and convection. Microvascular Research. 1989;**37**(1):77-104

[14] Anderson ARA, Chaplain MAJ, Newman EL, Steele RJC, Thompson AM. Mathematical modeling of tumour invasion and metastasis. Journal of Theoretical Medicine. 2000;**2**(2): 129-154

[15] Iwata K, Kawasaki K, Shigesada N. A dynamical model for the growth and size distribution of multiple metastatic tumors. Journal of Theoretical Biology. 2000;**203**(2):177-186

[16] Benzekry S, Gandolfi A, Hahnfeldt P. Global dormancy of metastases due to systemic inhibition of angiogenesis. PLoS One. 2014;**9**(1):e84249

[17] Baratchart E, Benzekry S, Bikfalvi A, Colin T, Cooley LS, Pineau R, Ribot EJ, Saut O, Souleyreau W. Computational modelling of metastasis development in renal cell carcinoma. PLoS Computational Biology. 2015;**11**(11):e1004626

[18] Stéphanou A, Mcdougall SR, Anderson ARA, Chaplain MAJ. Mathematical modelling of flow in 2D and 3D vascular networks: Applications to anti-angiogenic and chemotherapeutic drug strategies. Mathematical and Computer Modelling. 2005;**41**(10):1137-1156

[19] Wu J, Long Q, Xu S, Padhani AR. Study of tumor blood perfusion and its variation due to vascular normalization by anti-angiogenic therapy based on 3D angiogenic microvasculature. Journal of Biomechanics. 2009;**42**(6):712-721

[20] Soltani M, Chen P. Numerical modeling of interstitial fluid flow coupled with blood flow through a remodeled solid tumor microvascular network. PLoS One. 2013;**8**(6):e67025

[21] Zhao G, Yan W, Chen E, Yu X, Cai W. Numerical simulation of the inhibitory effect of angiostatin on metastatic tumor angiogenesis and microenvironment. Bulletin of Mathematical Biology. 2013;**75**(2):274-287

[22] Wu J, Ding Z, Cai Y, Xu S, Zhao G, Quan L. Simulation of tumor microvasculature and microenvironment response to anti-angiogenic treatment by angiostatin and endostatin. Applied Mathematics and Mechanics. 2011;**32**(4):437-448

[23] Cai Y, Wu J, Gulnar K, Zhang H, Cao J, Xu S, Long Q, Collins MW. Numerical simulation of solid tumor angiogenesis with endostatin treatment: A combined analysis of inhibiting effect of anti-angiogenic factor and micro mechanical environment of extracellular matrix. Applied Mathematics and Mechanics. 2009;**30**(10):1247-1254

[24] Baxter LT, Jain RK. Transport of fluid and macromolecules in tumors. (II) Role of heterogeneous perfusion and lymphatics. Microvascular Research. 1990;**40**:246-263

[25] Zhao G, Wu J, Xu S, Collins MW, Long Q, König CS, Jiang Y, Wang J, Padhani AR. Numerical simulation of blood flow and interstitial fluid pressure in solid tumor microcirculation based on tumor-induced angiogenesis. Acta Mechanica Sinica. 2007;**23**(5):477-483